Healthy Living

210 Habits and Advices That Help You Improve Health,
Transform Life & Live Healthy

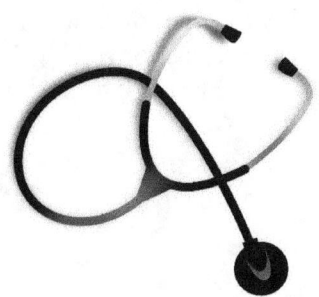

KiO Health

INTRODUCTION

Everyone has more-than-once suffered annoying health issues in our daily life. It is seen that some tips for everyday health treatment can be very useful for us to effectively avoid or deal with our frustrating health problems.

The environmental pollution nowadays, the busy working life of people and stresses in their daily life, all of them can lead to some senior health challenges. Some of the daily diseases people often catch are arthritis, heart disease, respiratory diseases, etc. Everyone knows that the pharmacists at the local area can dispense medicines for these health problems, but the truth is they can do a whole lot more besides. By being aware of these common health problems and how to deal with them, people can have a clearer control of their health, avoid some unexpected illnesses and have the right solution when it is needed by themselves.

With the diseases in the daily life, people can take very small actions to avoid them so efficiently. For example, to have a good state of health, sometimes all it needs is just making some healthy lifestyle choices, like stopping smoking and going on a diet to lose weight, etc. These actions are simple, but they can help you avoid senior health risks. Besides, you also need to be physically active and eat a healthy diet.

This project will let you take instant action to live a healthier life and get your very best state of health. It puts almost all health information needed in a basic level in the palm of your hands, supporting you with a complete control over every health decision in the daily life. Created by the credible health resources, this project can help you learn how to live better with any basic diseases. It makes getting healthy easier than ever, with easy tips, bottom-line advice from top experts, and riveting personal stories from people just like you.

TABLE OF CONTENTS

Chapter 1: How to deal fast with daily health problems

Almost instructions in this book aim to help you prevent or deal with some common diseases: how to avoid cardiovascular disease, how to give up smoking to prevent cancer, how to release stress which often results in high blood pressure affecting brain blood vessels negatively, how to keep control of alcohol taken in to prevent cirrhosis. Besides, this document will give you a large range of knowledge related to other diseases. Although some cases like belching, pain in the chest, back aches, asthenia, epistaxis, fever are not so serious to be taken to emergency, they still sometimes create intolerable discomfort to us.

This chapter will give 49 case studies on health problems occurring frequently in our daily life. It will also give you advice on how to deal with them properly.

1. How to avoid the headache and ease the pain

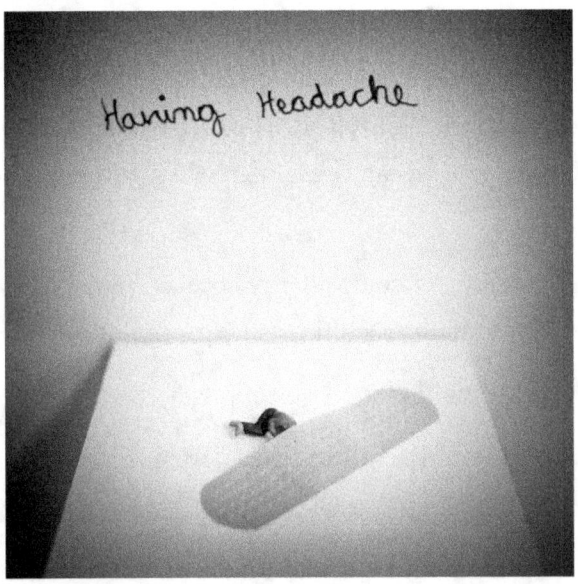

Many people have suffered from the headaches. In the Middle Ages, it is believed that the reason of the headaches is Satan entering our brains, so, they need to punch a small hole in our brains to get out. Fortunately, nowadays, the causes are discovered and doctors can give us the right treatment on the headache.

There are many symptoms of the headache, such as hypertension causing high pressure on brain's blood vessels, muscle's tension on some areas like face, neck, vertex that creates extreme pain especially on the forehead, temples and nape. The causes can be one of these cases: insomnia, tension on nerve resulting from busy working, taking charge of a huge amount of responsibilities, reading books constantly for a long time and so on.

A headache is often experienced by busy housewives who take care of so many household tasks and do so hard till getting exhausted. They can get tingling on temples, pain in half-brain and sometimes have symptoms of nausea, vomiting, vision limitation, dizziness or tinnitus.

The headaches from sinus can create pain in the face, on the forehead, in the area below forehead and in the middle area between forehead and cheeks, nasal bridge. Nasal inflammation and rheum can cause pain when patients press on the area of inflammation.

The causes can be catching a cold, allergy to a certain types of pollen, some problems of respiratory systems resulting from air pollution.

To relieve the pain, you should take these actions:

- Rest in a quiet and dark room (windows closed with curtains taken down), closed your eyes.

- Use your thumb to do massage from ear-zone to nape (the part below the skull), gently do massage on temples.

- Showers under warm water.

- Put a towel soaked in cold water on your eyes.

- Taking a dose of aspirin (those who have serious stomach ulcer must not do this because it can lead to dangerous stomach bleeding).

- Follow the guidelines in chapter 6 about methods of relaxation, such as keeping sitting quietly, doing meditation, and taking deep breath.

To prevent you from the headache, you should:

- Pay attention to your own body state to understand your periodical headache, frequently update news to get informed of time and place of epidemic cases as quick as possible.

- Get to know the headache symptoms to diagnose the disease.

- Should not eat a certain types of food which can easily cause the headaches to hypersensitive persons, such as:

+ Banana

+ Coffee and food with caffeine components.

+ Chocolate

+ Lemon, vinegar.

+ Salted meat.

+ MSG.

+ Dried lamb

+ Onions, garlic.

+ Red wine.

+ Yogurt

*Note: you should go to doctors if you have a constant headache for a long time or have an abnormal pain which has never been experienced before.

2. How to deal with fever?

It is not always the case that catching fever means you getting health problems. Many people at healthy state have body temperature of more or less than 37°C. But if oral reaches 37.2°C then you are surely having a fever.

Our body temperature is often at low lever in the morning and at high level in the afternoon or evening. Rectal temperature is usually higher than oral temperature by 0.3°C.

Taking oral temperature right after drinking hot water can make you mistakenly thought that you are having a fever. Your body temperature can increase due to the following reasons:

- Wearing too many clothes

- Doing exercise or moving so hard

- Hot and humid weather

- Increase or decrease of hormones (after ovulation, women's body temperature is often higher than normal).

If body temperature measured ranges from 37.2°C to 37.7°C or reaches higher number, you are surely having a fever. You need to go to the doctor if these cases happen to you:

- A less-than-6-month child gets high body temperature.

- If the child's oral temperature or rectal temperature remains high at 38.3°C or 38.8°C respectively during 48 hours.

- The same case is seen with adults, but the timing is 5 days. Additionally, there can be some symptoms such as a stiff neck, pain in the chest, vomiting, having diarrhea, lurching, rashing, coughing, having earache.

Fever with body temperature of less than 40°C is accepted as a normal fever. If the body temperature is higher than 40°C for a long time, then it is necessary to take a treatment.

To reduce body temperature, you should:

- Drink water or juice. Wipe your body with a cloth soaked in cool water of 21ºC.

- Take a dose of aspirin or acetaminophen suitable for your age once in every 3-4 hours (those who are under 19 years old with stomach injury should not do this).

- Relax, do not move so much.

- Do not wear so many clothes either cover yourself with a too thick blanket.

- Avoid strong movements.

3. Dandruff on the scalp

This case is harmless. This is a common skin disease when the sweat glands makes some spots on the head become greasy and makes white skin flakes easily slough off. There are even the cases with sloughed off skin flakes on eyebrows. The flakes fall down on the surfaces of the ears, the neck, on the nape and on the back area. The reason for this case is still unknown, but this symptom can be hereditary or can be the result of these phenomena:

- Stress, nervous tension.

- Not washing your hair frequently with soap.

- People having so much oiled sweat.

- Influence from the changing weather (too hot, too cold, too humid or too dry). The best thing to do here is to always wash your hair with shampoo.

Note when washing your hair:

- Slightly scratch the scalp to get rid of the dandruff, but be careful to not injure the skin.

- Use the shampoo which contains selenium sulfide to avoid dandruff

In serious cases, you need to go to a doctor to be prescribed with skin medicines which have cortisone ingredient.

4. Eight ways to deal with insomnia

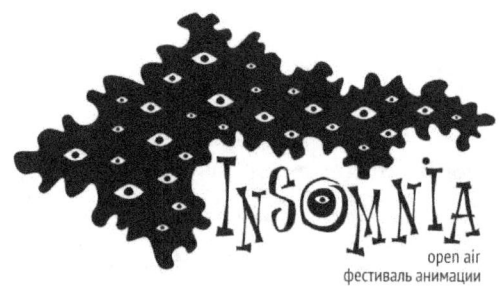

open air
фестиваль анимации

Have you ever suffered insomnia? If the answer is yes, then you don't have to worry so much, because it's a common case of many people. There's approximately 30 million American have this problem each day.

People suffering from insomnia can sleep a little bit when they start to go to bed. In the midnight or at the dawn, they wake up and could not fall asleep again. In fact, it is not that they can not sleep, they just get enough sleeping. However, if this phenomenon annoyed you for more than three weeks, then it needs you to take action.

Here are some applicable methods:

- Do not drink coffee, tea after lunch. Should stay away from chocolate, cola and other drinks which contains stimulants.

- Don't take a nap at noon, don't take a short nap at anytime even for a moment - it can affect your night-time sleep.

- Before sleeping, take a hot shower to relax muscles.

- Read books or do something repeatable, with no effort of thinking, such as knitting.

- Should not listen to the radio either watch television, these entertainment activities will make you have a heavier insomnia.

- Prepare a comfortable space to sleep which is quiet, with dim light. The bedroom should be prepared with clean blanket, pillow and bedspreads, with moderate temperature which is not hot either cold.

- Once you are on the bed, do not think about works anymore, just get the peace of mind to sleep.

- Establish a healthy daily routine, do the repeated series of actions which are locking doors, closing windows, brushing teeth and reading a story before going to bed.

- Count slowly before sleep as a hypnotized person. Think of blurred, boring and repeated images.

If you try to follow these methods in 3 weeks but you still can not sleep, you should go to a doctor to get the right treatments, and you can even get a neurological doctor or a psychology doctor if it's needed.

5. Pinkeye

In a morning, when you wake up and prepare to welcome a new day, you suddenly notice a discomfort from bulging and hassle eyelids. Looking in the mirror, you see your puffy eyes, the reddish pupils are filled with yellow rust. Then you are having pinkeye. Pinkeye is an inflammation inside the pupils, the upper and lower eyelids.

The cause of pinkeye can be one of these cases:

- The reaction of the eyes to some pollens, dust, animal's fur, dirty water or liquid cosmetics. Germs causing pinkeye generates rust in the eyes. In these two cases, take eye drops as prescriptives by the doctor. Covering eyes with a gauze impregnated with antibiotics. Pinkeye will end after 2, 3 days of treatment.

- A virus generated with flu and cold can also cause pinkeye. This virus creates less rust but makes you weep more. This case takes from 14 to 21 days to be cured.

Here are some treatments:

- Never use your hands to touch the eyes. If you want to wipe your eyes, you must use a clean towel.

- Close your eyes and grab a towel dipped in warm water to put on the eyes, 5 minutes for once. This will help you partially remove the eye rust.

- Use a dropper to drop your eyes. The eye drop will help you feel less itchy.

- Stop doing makeup with all kinds of lipstick, powder, artificial eyelashes. Do not share these makeup tools with others.

- Do not use bandages, gauze, cloth to cover your eyes. This can create more contamination on your eyes.

- Stop using magnifying glasses (glasses of watchmakers or jewelers).

- Always use separated hand towel, do not share with anyone. Pinkeye can be easily spread from person to person by hand contact and hand towel.

You need to go to a doctor if you do not get better after 2-3 days, if you have soreness in the eyes or often catch dazzling light when looking.

6. Hordeola

Hordeola can be caused by the inflammation of a small circuit in the eyelid. Hordeola can start from a bulging dot, then can develop into a red bead causing pain in the eyes. Before catching hordeola, you can have some of the following symptoms:

- Itchy eyelids

- Reddish eyelids

- Feeling bulging

- Feeling abnormal when touching. Initially, the wart emerges in the eyes in shape of a small yellow top with pus inside, then gradually grows into a larger yellow dot and breaks off.

If you have hordeola, you should:

- Put on the eyes a medical gauze soaked in warm water from 3 to 4 times a day, from 5 to 10 minutes for once.

- Avoid dirt getting in the eyes.

- Do not touch in the area having wart, even though you want to squeeze out immediately.

- Most of the cases can be treated at home, the wart is usually removed after 1-2 days of treatment. If the case does not get better after that time, you need to see a doctor to take more antibiotics following the prescription.

7. Eye fatigue because of sitting in front of the computer screen for a long time

Those who work with computers in the office usually complain about having tired eyes, back pain, aching shoulders and nervous tension.

Even though the computer screen does not emit harmful rays, but the situation of long-time sitting in one position, looking at an unchanged kind of dim light and keeping eyes on the tiny text can cause the typical diseases for people working in the office. Those who have to work with computer as a daily routine can reduce the negative impact of the computer by the following methods:

a. To protect your eyes:

- We should put the computer far away from the window to avoid direct light from outdoor or reflected light on the screen. The light shining down from the ceiling should be put behind a frosted glass. Additionally, you should add an anti-glare panel in front of the screen. You should put documents related to your work nearby when working with the computer. People often put documents on a shelf for easy reading.

- The angle created by the screen surface and the line from the eyes to the screen is about 10° to 15° (1/3 of the right angle).

- Keep the screen clean.

- Pay attention to blink your eyes several times to avoid your eyes from getting dried.

- Go checking eyes frequently and let your doctor know you are an officer working with computer as a daily routine. When you work, you should not wear makeup tools for the eyes such as eyelashes and stained glasses. Bifocals lenses are not suitable for working with computer because the second lenses are created to look straight on the books, they are not suitable for the angle of the eyes and the screen.

- If the screen's images are blurred or tuck, you should fix your computer immediately to avoid eye fatigue.

b. When having an eye fatigue or a headache, you should:

- Use chairs having suitable height for the vision on the screen.

- Leave the computer for a while, take a walk from 1 to 2 hours.

- Should have regular breaks during the work to do a number of exercises for the neck, shoulders and back. For example:

+ Tilt your head to the left and the right, back and forth, then move your head around the neck.

+ Push your shoulders up, down and then rotate them.

+ In standing or sitting position, crouch down to the forwards, to the right side, to the left side and then rotate the whole body.

8. Tinnitus

In the United States, there are about 36 million people suffering from tinnitus. In both day and night, at work and at rest, they always feel annoying whistle or crunching sound in the ears. Among them, about 7 million people have heavy cases, most of them are old people.

Like a toothache, tinnitus is not a disease but a symptom of a number of issues which need to be cared about. There are some reasons for tinnitus:

- Ears clogged because of earwax

- Food of medicine allergies

- Having inflammation in the middle of the ear.

- Abnormal phenomenon in cerebrovascular

- Abnormal phenomenon or a damage on the auditory nerve, because of hearing the loud and constant noise frequently.

- Diabetes

- Brain tumor

- Natural aging process

Tinnitus usually affects the ability to hear (unclear hearing or even hearing nothing), but does not lead to deafness.

When going to a doctor to check tinnitus, the doctor usually checks the whole system of Ear - Nose - Throat

To mitigate or eliminate tinnitus:

- Do not sit in front of the speaker of the radio or cassette to avoid loud sound. Avoid continuous sound.

- Use machines avoiding tinnitus. This looks like a music device, is often worn on the ear. This machine regularly emits a light sound wave to avoid outside noise. When wearing, people can hear other people talk as usual.

- Specialist can guide you through some exercises to relax the nerve to neglect the buzz in the ears.

- Exercise to enhance the blood circulation.

9. How to deal with epistaxis

Epistaxis or nosebleed is often seen in children. This symptom is caused by a small wound or cut on the blood vessels inside the nose, because of cold weather, allergies or dry weather that makes the nasal membranes be dried and then cracked.

The majority of the cases are terminated quickly. A small number of bleeding case can last long because the wound is deep inside the nose, and it is a common for adults because:

- Vascular sclerosis in the nose

- High Blood Pressure

- Regularly take anticoagulants

- Vascular diseases.

- Pimples in the nose.

Epistaxis cases often last from 10 to 15 minutes. If after that time, the case is not better, then you need to see a doctor to know the right disease and get the right treatment.

The normal cases of epistaxis can be treated by these method:

1. Sitting with back leaning on the chair, facing upward with the skyward nose.

2. Using your thumb and forefinger to squeeze slightly in the middle of your nose.

3. Breathing by your mouth in 10-15 minutes.

4. Using a gauze soaked in cold water to put on the nose.

5. During the time of 24 hours after the nosebleed, when you lie, put your head on high pillow to make sure the nose's position is always higher than the heart's position.

6. In that 24 hours, avoid carrying heavy goods, do not make heavy movements, avoid stress and hard work.

10. How to deal with impetigo in the mouth rim

Nothing is as annoying as impetigo in the mouth. A white blisters with red border around the mouth rim will make everyone pay attention to you. Even more, it is painful when you speak or eat and it makes you be not able to open your mouth. They slightly open the mouth for being polite while you do it because of the pain. Impetigo is very difficult to treat. Once you have it, you often have to wait for it to remove by itself.

Impetigo is repeated regularly, because the virus of this disease does not disappear forever. After causing impetigo, they often hide away inside our body and wait for another opportunity to show up again.

They often show up when we have a fever, a cold, a toothache, an eczema or when women have period.

First, we have the discomfort in the mouth rim. Look closely in the mirror, you will see a group of blistering nodules as like you are burnt, they are surrounded by a red or pink trim. Within 2 weeks, those red nodules dry into thin flakes, then you are cured.

To prevent impetigo, you should:

- Avoid negative emotional effects and overthinking situation

- Limit your exposure to sunlight. If it is necessary, apply a protective skin cream such as zinc oxide cream on the lips

- Avoid touching people with no impetigo

- Wash your hands to prevent the spread of the disease

To relieve the pain, you should:

- Put a gauze soaked in cold water on the area of disease

- Drink cold water

- Do not prick the injured area

- You can use painkillers such as aspirin, acetaminophen.

- If you have a severe pain, the doctor may give you medication known as Zovirax Acyclovir.

11. Avoid halitosis

Many people get upset because of halitosis. Standing close to other people to talk with them is very inconvenient. Having halitosis can be a symptom of many diseases.

- Slight smell of fruit in mouth can be a symptom of diabetes.

- Ammonia smell can prove renal insufficiency.

- Fish smell can be a symptom of liver weakness.

Furthermore, smelly mouth can be caused by diseases related to teeth, mouth, gum, throat and lungs, it also can be the result of the flu, hemorrhagic gastric area. Some foods can also be the causes, such as onion, garlic, volatile oil, a number of protein-rich foods.

Dentists often pay attention to the tooth track and the gum. Tracks in the teeth is the capacity for fermented foods. When having a gingivitis, blood pouring from the teeth's root can lead to smell.

Because there are many causes of halitosis, you should go to a dentist to get proper treatment for the disease. If there is no serious disease, we can take some actions to avoid halitosis:

- Careful brushing after meals. Note to brush the teeth's track.

- Scraping the tongue to get out the white residue on the tongue

- No smoking

- Rinsing after brushing your teeth everyday

- Go to a dentist to check your teeth and gum once in every 6 months.

12. Treatment for sore throat in the larynx

Sore throat is a common disease of politicians, actors and teachers, because they have to talk so much. Many sports force people to scream out loud such as jockey and basketball also make people have sore throat.

Air pollution, a lot of smoke from cigarette can also be the causes of this disease. When your throat hurts, your voice is weak, sometimes it is difficult to talk or in some cases, you even cannot talk. Sore throat can be accompanied with some phenomena of fever, cough, difficulty swallowing.

In such cases, if you continue smoking, drinking, talking outside the cold weather, singing, shouting, you will make the disease worse. Normally, you have to avoid talking in at least 2 days.

If the illness lasts longer than a week and there are some emerging phenomena such as fever, hemoptysis, yellow or brown sputum, you should go to the doctor immediately.

In common cases, the disease can be treated at home as it is mentioned bellow:

- Avoid saying, use body language if it is needed

- Speak slightly if you need to talk

- Open the air conditioner to warm your room.

- Drink plenty of warm water (honey tea is very good).

- Take shower or soak in hot water.

- Do not smoke and stay away from smoking areas.

- Take medicine for sore throat.

- Use aspirin to reduce pain if it is necessary.

13. Hiccup

The cause of the hiccup is the diaphragmatic which lies between the chest and the abdomen having "cramps". In normal cases, this phenomenon doesn't last long. But it is possible to shorten the time of hiccup in several ways:

- Swallow 1 teaspoon of dried sugar

- Use your fingers to hold the tongue and pull out.

- Tilt the neck backwards, stop breathing for a moment, mentally count from 1 to 10, snort and then drink a cup of water.

- Put a paper bag on your nose and mouth, breathe in and out several times.

- Swallow a small ice cube.

- Use a cotton swab, wipe the inside of the palate

- Eat slowly a piece of dried cake

- Drink a glass of water quickly.

The hiccups lasting long can be a symptom of heart disease or stomach disease, so, you should go to a doctor.

In the section number 12, we talked about sore throat. Because the larynx in the throat is injured, so, you suffer pain in your throat. In this article, we mention the sore throat caused by a virus or bacteria.

The bacteria causing sore throat are Streptococcus. It also causes fever, a headache, sore throat and lymphadenopathy in the neck. In a contrary, if a sore throat is caused by virus, we will not see the above symptoms. However, many cases of bacterial sore throat in children can make doctors confused because of no symptoms seen. If we do not take timely treatment, this disease can lead to some serious cases such as nephritis, heart failure and cases of abscess. Therefore, doctors need to diagnose exactly what the reason of the sore throat is, to decide whether the patient needs to take antibiotics or not. A dose of antibiotics can be prescribed for a 10-day treatment.

We can deal with sore throat by the following methods:

- Rinse with warm salted water.

- Drink plenty of warm water, soup, warm tea with honey.

- Heat the bedroom.

- Do not smoke.

- Avoid eating spicy foods or stimulants such as pepper and curry powder

- Eat sugar or candy.

- If you have a fever, you can use medications such as aspirin or acetaminophen (acetamol). Note: if you are less than 20 years old or having stomach ailments, you should not use aspirin.

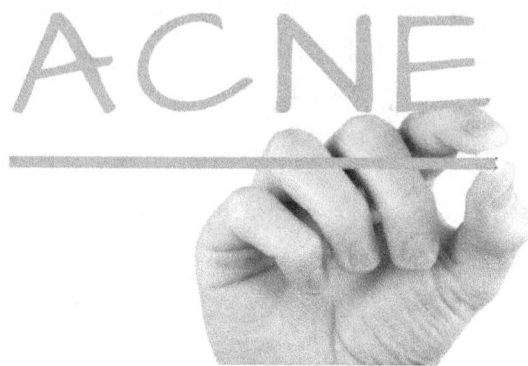

What will happen when a teenage young girl or a teenage young boy starts to pay attention to friends of the opposite gender? And what happens if the acne appears at that time? Acne of white, red or black color and the small pimples in the areas of shoulders, back, neck and especially on the face will make people upset. This phenomenon can continue to occur even when people has gone through the teenage. It is not the result of eating more much fat foods or chocolate as many people mistakenly believe.

The cause of acne is the increasing amount of sex hormones at puberty. The slime on the surface of the skin creates acne. The sebaceous glands under the skin is clogged, then they create the shelter for bacteria causing acne.

There can be some other reasons:

- The increase of hormones of the endocrine glands during the period or pregnancy of women.

- The perfume or facial oil can form a lubricant layer on the skin.

- The stressful situation.

- Foods which contain a lot of iodine, such as asparagus, kelp, white onions.

- Cooking and making ingredients of oil attached on the skin.

- Regular contacting with detergents such as creosote.

- Sleeping on one side that makes a side of you face be pressed for a long time

- Use of drugs for birth control, avoiding muscle contraction or drugs with lithium ingredient.

Acne will dive away after a while. But we should also know how to protect your skin during the time of having as stated bellow:

- Keeping skin clean by washing the face with soap several times a day. Using a clean towel to wipe your face and massage in about 1-2 minutes.

- Towel used to wipe face has to be clean. After wiping face, you have to wash the towel and dry it because the bacteria can attach to the towel and grow in wet condition, then attack the skin through the pores.

- Asking specialists to buy the soap used for skin with acne.

- No squeezing, pricking and touching the acne. Doing so can cause skin infections and form scars.

- You can use topical medications have ingredient of benzoyl peroxide. Note: some people with reactive skin should not use.

- After hard movements, you should wipe the sweat from the skin to make the pores open.

- Washing your head with soap for at least 2 times per week to clean the mucus which can affect the skin on the forehead, in the neck and the shoulders.

- Avoid letting your hair touch your face

- With men, before shaving, you should wipe your face by a towel soaked in warm water. Shaving beards along the side of beard growing can avoid scratching the skin.

- Avoid expose to the sunlight a lot.

- Avoid hot lights shinning on the skin.

- Avoid using oils, creams which can form adhesive greasy layer on the skin.

- If the skin have more acne than usual, you should go to a doctor.

16. Catching a cold

Every day, there are about 80 million Americans having a cold with symptoms of coughing, stuffy and runny nose (rhinorrhea). A person often catch a cold 3-4 times a year. If you do not often catch a cold, then it is a very lucky, because a cold caused by viruses can be spread so easily.

Firstly, you can have the stuffy, a little water can flow from your nose, you can sneeze or have a slight fever (possibly up to 39ºC), you can also have sore throat and coughing. The cold often lasts after 3 to 7 days.

A cold can spread from person to person through the air by coughing and sneezing. There are studies showing that patients' hands are often attached by nasal mucus after coughing or sneezing because the patients usually use hand to cover their mouths and noses or wipe their mouths and noses with a tissue. When you have a cold, you should avoid it spread to others, by these following actions:

- Frequently wash your hands.

- When you cough, sneeze or have a runny nose, you have to take a tissue to cover your mouth and nose, then fold it back.

- Avoid shaking hands and touching others. The coins and money of the patients can also be the causes of the cold spreading.

Patients should:

- Take a rest, especially in the case of a fever.

- Drink plenty of hot or cold water. Water can erase the sputum in the throat.

- Take aspirin or acetaminophen to relieve pain and tenderness. Note: people of 19 years old or younger should not take aspirin.

- Rinse your mouth with warm salted water, drink tea with honey and lemonade or eat candies to reduce the negative effect of sore throat.

- Steam.

- Chicken soup (with small chicken) can be a useful treatment.

17. Sinusitis

Sinus lies in the path of air moving through the nose into the lungs. When going through the sinuses, the air is warmed up. If the sinus are infected, you will have a stuffy nose, have a headache or cough. Sometimes, the headache can make you cannot sleep. If you smoke and have an abnormal phenomenon in the nose, the symptoms can be more serious, such as:

- A headache.

- Stuffy nose, nasal dripping in dark yellow color.

- Pain on the forehead and on the upper side of the face, in the nose area and on the upper jaw.

- Pain often recur when turning over your body while lying, it can temporarily stop when sitting up.

- Fever.

To soothe the pain, inhale cold air, or take these actions:

- Drink plenty of water to ventilate the nose.

- Take aspirin or acetaminophen to relieve pain.

- Take nasal drop

Note:

- Do not give aspirin to people aging 19 years old or less.

- Do not take nasal drop for more than 3 days, because this will make the nose get used to medicine, make you have stuffy nose whenever there is no medicine.

- Do not use nasal tubes used by others to prevent the spread of the disease.

- If home treatment does not work, you should go to the doctor with special skills for ear - nose - throat problems. So, if it is necessary, you can take antibiotics.

In severe sinus cases, you may have to go through a minor operation.

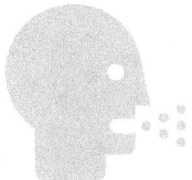

Each year, up to 50,000 people in the US die because of pneumonia which starts from the flu.

Cold and flu are almost the same, but we can distinguish them by some noticeable differences. People having a cold usually begin with a runny nose, sneezing, mild discomfort.

People who have a flu lose energy faster. They can turn from the healthy state to the exhaustion state right in one hour.

A cold rarely attacks the lungs, but a flu can create complication and lead to pneumonia.

People catching a cold can still try to work, but people having a flu have no strength to go to work.

Therefore, if we are struck down quickly, we are having a flu. These symptoms can be accompanied:

- Dry cough

- Sore throat

- The serious headaches

- Aching muscles

- Feeling so tired

- Getting chills

- Body temperature can be up to 40 ° C

- Eyestrain.

The symptoms which are most obvious to us are getting very tired and getting serious aches (sore muscles). Catching a cold will not lead to these symptoms.

Actually, there is no drug to immediately stop the flu. You have to let it go away by itself. The purpose of medicine is to reduce the pain and prevent disease from development and complications. Normally, we can self-treat at home. But, if you breathe difficultly, cough, have yellow or green phlegm, then you need to go to a doctor, because the flu can have complication and cause pneumonia.

If it is a mild flu, you need to rest to save energy for the body to fight against the influenza virus. Besides, we should follow the following instructions:

- Drink plenty of hot water to ventilate pulmonary- nasal system and offset the amount of water lost due to sweating.

- Rinse your mouth with salted water.

- Eat hard candy to help relieve the sore throat.

- Do not avoid coughing because coughing helps ventilate the tubes in the lungs and send the mucus outward. If the nose sputum have blood, you should go to a doctor.

- Abstain from drinking milk, do not eat cheese and other foods made from butter or milk in 2 days because they have the effect of creating the mucus in the nose and clogging throat.

- Wash hands frequently, especially before eating to avoid spreading the flu to others.

- Drink a dose of aspirin (people aging 19 or less should not take aspirin).

If home treatment do not help you feel better, you should go to a doctor.

In many areas, the government organize frequent flu injections for those who age over 65. In every case of a flu spreading, you should update the news frequently to be timely informed of the prevention actions.

19. Asthma

Do you know anything about asthma? Regularly, there are 10 million Americans having asthma. When they cough, they wheeze hard and it feels like their lungs are shrinking. Asthma can be the result of physical causes but not psychological causes. Once you have asthma, the agitations of psychology such as fear, anxiety and anger can create stress and make it worse, although they are not the causative factors. When a patient has an asthma but does not take remedies promptly, the patient may die.

What does an asthma differ from other diseases of the respiratory organs? The cause of asthma is simply the spasm of muscle in the air pipes to the lungs, it makes the air pipe narrow and makes the patient cannot breathe because of the lack of oxygen. Some cases bellow have negative impacts and can lead to seizures:

- Breathing air with pollen, dust, mold, smoke, dust and dirt.

- Eating or drinking substances which the body easily reacts on.

- Being too nervous or emotional.

- Working so hard or heavy movements.

- Exposure to respiratory diseases.

Asthma can be mild or serious, the progression of the disease is often complex that you may need a doctor to help you take right treatment and medicine.

However, the patients can take care by themselves by the following guidelines:

- Drink plenty of water every day (2-3 liters/day).

- Get rid of the strange smell from your house, especially in the bedroom or workplace.

- Avoid using animal-fur pillows, replace them by synthetic pillows.

- Do not smoke.

- Avoid places having pollen.

- When going outdoors, cover your nose and your mouth, especially when the weather is cold, to warm the air before the air goes into your body.

- If you have breathing problems when working, you must stop working immediately.

- Avoid foods or medicines having sulphide ($-SO_3$) in the ingredients. SO_3 is often found in wine.

- When you have seizures, you must sit up but not lie down

- The drugs and immediate treatment should be put near the patient to apply immediately when it is needed

- You have to figure out whether you have allergy to aspirin or not. You should use acetaminophen instead of aspirin.

Doctors often prescribe these medications for asthma patients:

- Bronchodilator - a medication for drinking or spraying into the throat to make you breathe easier.

- Steroids - to avoid body reactions to strange substances

- Cromolyn sodium for inhalation to prevent seizures. Once there is a seizure, this medication will not work anymore.

20. Fever in the season of hay

A doctor in the 19th century named this disease because each time he walked on a house with dried-grass roof, he got sick. Today, we get used to calling the disease 'fever in the season of hay', even though the disease is not related to the dried grass.

Many people suffer from this disease in the spring. There are people having this disease all year round with the symptoms: runny eyes, runny noses, getting congested, choking. The main cause of the disease is the body's response to the air pollution.

Here are some tips:

- Clean the house to get rid of all the weed leaves, branches, seeds and moldy items, do not let your dog take garbage, bones and defecate in the house.

- Close the doors and windows in the season of pollen and in the weather having high-humidity air.

- Use air conditioning to warm bedroom and filter the air, the objects in the bedroom have to be clean as always.

- The rooms in the house must be cleaned frequently.

- Wash blankets as frequently, keep them always clean because it directly exposes to the nose and the mouth.

- Avoid taking blankets, clothing outside for drying because the pollen and dust can easily stick to them.

If the above actions do not work, you should go to a doctor to take additional drugs such as:

- Anti-histamine (antihistamines) to limit the reaction of the body against strange substances. This drug should be used 30 minutes before going out.

- Decongestants (drinking or spraying), you should not use nose drops more than 3 days to not make the body get used to taking medicine. If the body get used to medicine, you will have the disease whenever you do not take the medicine.

- Eye drops.

In addition, doctors can prescribe some drugs bellow:

- Cromolyn sodium and steroids.

- Immune drug.

- Examination of skin samples to know what kind of substance the skin reacts on.

- Injections to avoid body reaction.

21. Bronchitis

If you cannot stop coughing, the cough seems to rise from toes to the upwards, makes you shake the whole body, then you are having a bronchial infection which is also known as bronchitis.

They distinguish acute bronchitis and chronic bronchitis basing on the duration of the disease and its consequences.

Acute bronchitis is often caused by bronchial mucous membranes attacked by viruses, infections or environmental factors (eg cigarette smoke), causes swelling and irritation on the bronchial system. Bronchitis often leads to inflammation or other infections on the airways. The disease may take from 3 days to 3 weeks to end.

The early symptom of acute bronchitis is coughing, having chills, slight fever, sore throat and pain in muscle.

Treatments:

- Steam nose by inhaling warm water steam (using tools or machines may help you breathe better).

- Put medicine into the throat by the throat spray.

- Take antibiotics.

- Take aspirin or acetaminophen to deal with fever and pain.

- Use a drug to stimulate coughing to get rid of mucus.

- Take a rest

- Drink a lot of water.

- Do not smoke.

To fully recover, sometimes it takes up to 1 month. If after 1 week of treatment, you do not get better, please go to a doctor, because the disease can be transformed into pneumonia.

People with chronic bronchitis often cough a lot and have more phlegm, the disease can last from 2 months to 2 years, this case is mostly seen in men. The disease often damage alveolar system that it can affect the exhaling- inhaling function of the lungs and negatively affect the respiratory system.

The symptoms of chronic bronchitis are:

- Short breath when inhaling.

- Short resting time between breaths.

- Coughing with thick yellow phlegm.

Those who easily have chronic bronchitis are often the people living in the air pollution in the industrial zones. They can be workers who are frequently exposed to metal dust, dust from cotton yarn and those who smoke.

To prevent chronic bronchitis, you should:

- Avoid polluted places. If it is necessary, there should be tapes covering the nose, mouth.

- Do not go out the streets during the time of heavy air pollution.

- Use expectorant medicine, tracheostomy medicine and antibiotics when you get sick, follow the guidance of the pharmacist.

- If the disease lasts longer than a week, you need to go to a doctor to consider whether the disease is turned into a pneumonia or not.

22. Pain in esophagus terminal

In the United States nowadays, there are many diseases are called wrongly, but people do not change the name because the names have become so popular. For example, after a good meal, you could feel a burning pain in the lower chest on the left side, in the heart area. The Americans call it as "heart burn". In fact, there is no issue related to the heart, the disease's cause is the digestive juices in the stomach having so much acidic that moves upwards to the tube connecting the esophagus with the stomach. This area is just behind the heart, this is the phenomenon of pain in esophagus terminal.

Gastric (stomach) has an inner layer of protection. So, you do not feel the effects of acid on your stomach, except from those who have stomach ulcer, their esophagus part has no protective layer. Then, when having acid on the digestive juices, they will feel the burning pain immediately.

Here are some the reasons:

- Eating plenty of foods cause indigestion.

- Eating fast.

- Eating so much chocolate, garlic, onions and spicy foods like peppermint.

- Smoking after a meal.

- Drinking so much coffee and alcohol.

- Taking aspirin

- Having hernia which is a malformation of the stomach, when there is an abnormal organ part moving up next to the esophageal system, making digestive juices inside the stomach move into the esophagus. Nearly a half of the whole number of more-than-60-year-old people have this situation.

So, here are some advice on how to deal with the pain:

- Siting with the straight back or standing up, walking back and forth for a while.

- Avoiding bending or lying, because doing so can make digestive juices flow into the esophagus.

- If you have a pain at night, quietly raise your head and put under your head a high pillow.

- Finding ways to lose weight, fat people and pregnant women easily have pain in the esophagus because the bulging stomach can put pressure on the esophagus.

- Avoiding overeating, eating easily digested foods.

- Drinking 1-2 teaspoons of diluted magnesium hydroxide, once in every 1-2 hours.

Note: people with heart diseases, kidney diseases, high blood pressure should ask doctors before using that anti-acid medicine.

- Drinking a glass of milk, milk does not have the function of neutralizing acid but it can ease the pain.

23. Constipation

Constipation is a common condition that affects people of all ages. It can mean that you're not passing stools regularly or you're unable to completely empty your bowel. People do not see it as a "disease" and other diseases, but who are constipated can feel very uncomfortable. The aim of these treatments is to make the bowel work in smooth condition:

- Eat more fruits and vegetables, because they have plenty of fiber substances. The fiber can absorb water, then the foods can become smaller when they pass the narrow path in the bowel. Therefore, the stools can easily move outside.

- Eat the breads made from whole grains and nuts.

- Drink a lot of water.

- Do exercise, so that the bowel can also do exercise in your stomach. When it is necessary, go to the toilet immediately, do not hold it back.

Note: the anti-acid medicines or medicine having iron ingredients can cause heavier constipation for those who already have constipation.

- You can ask your doctor to take medication to soften the stools.

If you apply the above treatments and see no positive results, take bowel medicines. Do not take bowel medicines immediately because it can make the bowel lose natural squeezing actions to move stools out. Using so much medicine can also makes the body lose the balance of metal compounds in the body.

Abusing douching can also lead to negative effect as mentioned above.

If you are constantly constipated, you should go to a doctor to know whether there are any different causes, such as:

- Some unsuitable medications you have taken.

- A number of health problems, such as hemorrhoids related to the anal sphincter, ineffective work of the thyroid and enteritis.

24. Deal with diarrhea

The diarrhea is in contrast to the constipation. It is also a common disease of us. In the minor case, the situation lasts in one or two days. However, the pain in the abdominal is unforgettable. The reasons for the diarrhea can be one of these cases:

- Being poisoned because of viruses, bacteria, eating or drinking contaminated stuff, especially on the road traveling to strange places.

- Eating out-date cakes.

- The digestive system has allergies.

- The abuse of medicines.

- Mental disorder.

- Allergy to some antibiotics like tetracyclines, cleocin, ampicillin.

- Enteritis.

- Symptoms of bowel cancer.

Diarrhea makes body lose water. Therefore, you need to drink plenty of water to compensate. This is essential, especially for children. The patients should eat soup, take in the broth, drink ginger water, take in some ice and drink boiled water.

Here are some things you should pay attention to:

- Just eat a few, in the first day, avoid eating solids.

- Eat bananas, rice porridge, apple juice and toast , these foods have good effect to harden the stools.

- When you get better, eat some snack and soft things, abstain from fat, oil, grease and protein.

- Do not eat much food having fibrous substance and breads made from grains or cereals.

- Avoid fruit, raw vegetables, cooled food in refrigerators, candy, coffee and hard food.

- Limit your activities to rest the bowel, can take in bismuth medicine.

If the situation lasts more than 72 hours and even if there are bloody stools, you need to go to a doctor for right treatments.

25. How to avoid flatulence

Flatulence is a normal case for everyone. But it cause too much inconvenience if the situation is heavy. The bacteria in the bowel turn foods into carbon dioxide and hydrogen. These pure gases does not smell, but when being mixed with some other gases such as hydrogen sulfide and waste substances, the smell is so heavy.

There are some foods making the digestive system generate gases more than other foods. We need to know them to avoid eating so much, especially before we go to meetings or dating. Those foods are some vegetables and fruits, such as:

- Some types of green-leave vegetables including cabbage

- Broccoli (soup Saul)

- Some types of green fruit.

- Some types of bean like peas, soybeans and so on.

- Pear

- Apple

- Peach

- Plum

- Onion

- Grape

- Popcorn

- Cheese

In the medicine which helps to avoid farting, people often use Simethicone which is also called as Mylicon.

When the abdominal part bulges out so much, we should think about the following issues:

- The digestive system does not work well with milk and dairy and fat foods.

- There is too much bacteria in the bowel.

- The contraction of the bowel in the normal state.

26. Urinary tract infection

On average, one in every 5 women have a urinary tract infection. Men are also susceptible, but less than women.

To understand this issue, we need to know the urinary system of the body including kidney, bladder (bladder), urinary tract kidney connected with bladder (ureters), the tube that carries urine from the bladder (urethra) to the outside.

In women, the urethra is very susceptible to infection because this is often touch because of friction during sex that causes the bacteria easily enter. Catheter infection can lead to inflammation in the kidneys. Therefore, after sex, people should pee immediately even though they feel no need. Such urination is purposed to expel the bacteria to the outside. The pregnant women who often have catheter pressed by the fetus and the uterus, people having not smoothly catheter (disfigurement) often get inflammation in the urinary system easier than others.

The symptoms of urinary tract infection can include:

- Always feel the urge to urinate.

- Urinate frequently with a small amount

- Feeling irritating in urinary system.

- Bloody urine.

- After urinating, the bladder still feels full.

- Lower abdominal pain (bladder) or both sides of the abdomen (kidney).

- Feel chills, have a fever, have a nausea, vomit (symptoms of inflammation of the kidneys).

If you have these symptoms, you should go to a doctor immediately. The longer, the more severe the disease. The doctor will take a urine sample to test and figure out the situation of the disease.

You have to take enough antibiotics prescribed by the doctor. Remember to take an enough dose, even though you can no longer see the symptoms in the middle of the medicine duration.

There are some of preventative methods:

- If you are a female, you need to clean and dry the pee hole and genitals after urination and after bathing.

- Drink a lot of water, urinate frequently because every time you do it, you are washing the urinary tube and sending the bacteria out.

- Do not try to hold back the want to urinate.

- After having sex, urinate immediately, even though you do not feel the need.

- Wear cotton underwear, avoid hot and humid materials which are suitable for bacterial growth.

- Women who are having the disease should avoid washing the genitals with the douching tools.

27. Avoid chibiain caused by cold weather

Each year, 10,000 Americans suffer from chibiain.

Looking at the outside effects, chibiain looks like herpes on the skin. In fact, the skin at that site could be frozen and destroyed. The skin areas which easily get chibiain are fingers, toes, earlobes, chin and nose tip.

Firstly, people feel the pain in the site of chibiain, and then those places bubble, blister and lose all sense.

Depending on whether the cold weather come slowly or suddenly, people can feel or cannot feel the chibiain. It is wrong if you want to put snow on the chibiain or soak the sore hands into the cold water. Instead, you need to:

- Soak your hands into the hot water from 38ºC to 40ºC and antibiotic solution, stop do so when you can feel again, the duration can take about 45 minutes.

- Go to the emergency room because chibiain can cause a tetanus infection.

To prevent the chibiain, you should:

- Wear several layers of pants, shirts and socks. Many layers of thin coat are better than a layer of thick coat because the air layer between the coat layers can heat and warm up the body very well.

- Avoid alcohol and smoking, alcohol can make your blood temperature decrease fast and tobacco can slow the blood flow, especially to the ending point of your body such as toes and fingers.

- When the outdoor temperature is too low and if it is accompanied with heavy wind, you should stay indoors.

28. Itchy feeling in the winter

In winter, people often feel itchy. The reason is the skin can be dried to the state of cracking and swelling.

To relieve the winter itch, you should think about how to retain moisture on the skin. Therefore, you should not bath several times a day because water and soap dissolves mucus which protects the skin. With old people, this mucus's amount will decrease. You should:

- Use slight soap.

- After taking shower, use a bath towel to cover your body rather than wipe your body.

- Avoid soaking your hands into hot water and detergent. If it is necessary, use protective gloves.

- Avoid sitting near the fireplace, use a spray machine to keep the moisture in the room.

29. Avoid heat rash

Heat rash is a skin disease occuring in the summer, especially in the tropical countries. It happens when many small blisters floating on the skin that makes rash on the hands, neck, armpits and back but there will be no rashes on the face. Hot weather, sensitive skin and getting fat are some conditions to have heat rashes.

To avoid heat rash, you should:

- Wear light-weight, thin and airy clothes.

- Sprinkle talcum powder on the spots which have heat rashes.

- Bath in cool water.

- Avoid hot, moist and dirty places and if it is possible, use air conditioning.

If you are in a cool place, the rash will get away by itself within 1-2 days.

30. Itchy feeling because of contacting with the tree's resin

A walk in the woods, on the grass to look canopy and listen to the birds always creates a lot of fun and day dreams. However, you should be careful because the dreamer will quickly dissipate if you suddenly feel all the body is getting itchy. The reason is that some plants generate resin which can cause itchy blisters on the skin.

In such cases, you should:

- Do the laundry with all the clothes. If clothes cannot be washed, you should hang them in front of or in an airy space in about 3 weeks.

- Shower with soap, use an alcohol-soaked swab to slightly apply on the itchy area, then clean the area with clean water.

The resin can cause itchy feeling in 2-3 days. If there are irritations, wash the area and cover it with calamine solution.

- You can use some medicines antihistamines such as diphenhydramine which is also known as benadryl.

- If the skin blisters continue to widespread, you can wash the area with a solution of soda slightly. Such washing can break the blisters but will stop the spreading.

- If the blisters still spread, especially in the mouth, eyes and genitals, you need to go to a doctor for right treatment. The prescribed medicine can be steroids which is to drink or to put on the itchy area.

31. How to deal with exanthema

After a delicious meal with special foods such as crab, shrimp and oysters, you can get rashes all over your body. These blisters are like mosquito bites, but in red groups emerging from the face, the body, the arms, the legs and the thighs, causing itchy feeling. This is exanthema. Exanthema can disappear after 24 hours but it can come back at anytime.

The causes of exanthema can be:

- Body hydrophobic against drugs such as aspirin fish, sunfa and penicillin.

- Cold weather.

- Fatigue or stress.

- Certain foods such as chocolate, almonds and tomatoes.

- Being poisoned

- The body reaction to some substances such as pollen, mold and chemical smell

- Being attacked by insects.

- The skin being scratched.

- Myositis.

We do not identify the cause of the rashes in many cases. However, the treatment or prevention of exanthema is necessary because the disease can lead to death in case of exanthema appearing in the tongue and throat areas that makes patients unable to breathe, or the rashes affecting the heart, lungs and digestible parts.

Once you have exanthema, you should follow the following instructions:

- No hot-water bath is applied, you can take a warm bath. High temperature can make the situation worse.

- Apply cold towels to the area of exanthema.

- Wear loose and airy clothes.

- Take a rest, try to relax the body and spirit.

- Ask your doctor to take antihistamines (Note: this drug causes drowsiness). Therefore, after taking the drug, you must not drive or engage in any activities that require quick reactions. Do not take aspirin because it can make the situation worse.

32. Deal with warts

Warts may make your hands and foots look ugly, but it is harmless. They can spread from person to person. They classify some types of wart:

- Shallow circular warts in hand in light black color, sometimes they grow in clusters with small dots surrounding a large dot.

- Deep warts with the root going deep into the skin, they usually appear on the soles of the foot that cause pain when you stand or walk. Therefore, the pressure on the foot should be eased by a buffer layer.

Deep warts are also contagious. Therefore, avoid direct touching the foot with warts. The shared bathroom is the place of easy disease spreading. When bathing, do not use barefoot to touch the floor and you should dry your feet immediately after a bath.

Some warts will disappear. Some can be treated with salicylic acid or lactic acid. When using this acid, you should be careful to not make acids stick to other areas, because acid can damage skin.

Doctors often treat warts by these methods:

- Using liquid nitrogen.

- Executing minor surgery for deep warts.

- Using lasers

- No burning with electric power because there will be scars.

33. How to prevent eczema

Allergic eczema usually appears in the form of small blisters, can have hard itchy scaly and irritation, in both children and adults. Eczema can be hereditary. People with asthma are often associated with eczema.

The following cases can cause more serious illness:

- Wear woolen or fur clothes.

- Sweat.

- Have nervous tension (Stress)

- Live in hot and humid places

- Eat eggs, seafood (crab, fish, snails …), milk and wheat foods.

- Exposure to these chemicals: the detergent, perfume, skin cream and pharmaceuticals.

It is difficult to treat eczema. Many patients live with it for a lifetime, the disease reduced at old age and then it is healed. However, we can ease the eczema by following actions:

- Bath little, avoid long baths, you should take a shower. If you use the bath tub, add bathing oil into the water.

- Take a warm bath.

- Do not use soap or just use a little soap when bathing.

- Avoid wearing woolen clothes

- After a shower, avoid applying on the skin the oily and perfumed liquid.

- Do not wear many clothes to cool the body.

- Avoid food, medicine and perfume causing allergies.

- Seriously avoid scratching, scratching will cause the skin injured, enable the skin to get infection.

34. Chickenpox

Chickenpox is a common case of children but sometimes they can also emerge from adults. This disease is spread to children, but not to adults. Virus only attacks adults of over 50 years old, in which case the immune system of them are particularly weak and they can potentially get a cancer.

The symptoms can be:

- Skin feeling itchy before getting chickenpox

- The red blisters appear and then disappear, usually appear on the back, on the two sides of the face, sometimes emerge in the eye area.

- Sometimes it is accompanied by a fever and feeling tired.

After 3 weeks, the chickenpox can disappear, but you can still feel sore on the skin after 1-6 months.

When the spots are dried or broken, you should:

- Do not put bandage on pimples, do not wear tight-fitting clothes.

- Rinse the dots but do not scratch.

- Apply towel soaked in cold water, calamine lotion or soda water on the chickenpox.

Note: if there is any dot in the eye, ask the doctor to take additional medicines and steroids medicine, especially in the case of infection.

35. Avoid stinging by insects

Camping under a tree, lying on the beach during summer days are so interesting. But how to avoid insect bites?

- Pack food and beverages carefully, especially sweets.

- Avoid using oils, skin creams with perfume.

- Do not wear colorful clothes, should choose clothes of white or a single color.

- Wear long clothes, cover hands and feet, don't go on barefoot

In case of being bitten by insects, you should:

- Gently pick the insect's stinger out, as soon as possible.

- Do not scratch or take the insect stinger by hand because the stinger can be poisonous. Doing so can cause the sting become more painful (with bees, they often left the poisonous stinger back on the skin after stinging).

- Wash the stinging area with soap.

- Use ice to press on the injured site to reduce pain and apply antihistamines on the skin.

- Taking aspirin or acetaminophen, together with antihistamines.

- If the insect stings in the mouth or on the tongue, you need to call emergency immediately because it can affect your respiration.

In almost cases, the stinging area is itchy, painful and irritated, but depending on the position, the body may react differently, it can grow from swelling into the state of breathlessness, increasing heartbeat, being fainted or death.

Therefore, you should base on the situation to decide whether you have to go to emergency. Going camping in remote area, you have to carry emergency drugs, including drugs that reduce the body's reaction, antibiotics and heart tonic. People having body reaction to the stings must prepare methods to take care of themselves.

36. What finger nails can tell about your health

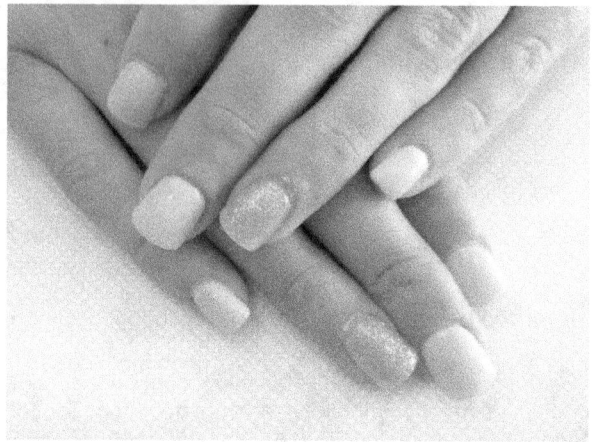

You've seen your fingers a thousand times, but have you ever thought whether the nails may reflect the state of health?

Nail roots have white spots with spoon shape shows that your body is lacking iron. Thin and brittle nails means the single glandular thyroid in the throat works inefficiently.

To keep the nails being nice which reflects your body's health, you should:

- Eat more fruits and vegetables, nuts, fresh meat and low-fat foods.

- Wear gloves to protect the hand when you have to touch chemicals and detergents.

- Clean the nails after working.

- Trim the epidermis in the corners of the fingers to avoid scratches in this section.

- Do not use nails to brick anything.

- Do not cut the nails too close to the flesh.

The table bellow will tell how nails reflect the health:

State of Nails	Possible health problems
crispy, brittle nails	Being soaked in a long time in hot water, poor health, lack of vitamin A, C, B6, calcium, iron, underactive thyroid.
uneven nails	Heart, lung weakness, symptoms of cancer, congenital weakness.
the surface is not smooth	Eczema, trauma or psoriasis.
not straight, undulating nails	Rheumatoid arthritis, kidney diseases, aging process, emphysema.
cracking	Allergy to substances of nails, iron deficiency, lack of red blood cells, pregnancy, psoriasis.
cracking on the tip	Long-time being soaked in the water, replacing nails.
there are white streaks having spoon shape	Inefficient working of endocrine gland activity (thyroid) and erythrocyte iron deficiency.

37. How to deal with the situation of getting tired

Although science and technology have helped us to accomplish many daily tasks, many still go to the doctor and complain: I get tired...

Each of us should know why we get tired and what is the cause? They often classify two types of fatigue: getting tired physically and getting tired mentally.

Many workers are often tired in the afternoon and can restore their health after a night's sleep: it's the kind of getting tired physically.

Tired people are usually tired mentally in the morning and they often get better in the afternoon. The cause of physical exhaustion can be one of these cases:

- Not enough eating and sleeping

- The amount of metal compounds in the blood is improper to the ratio of Na and K.

- Working in hot and humid environment.

- Anemia.

- Having prolonged influenza or cold.

- Being infected by Virus

- Some endocrine glands like the thyroid work inefficiently.

Causes of mental exhaustion can be:

- Taking charge of too much work, being so worried.

- Doing boring works.

- There is an unexpected event in the life (like divorce or retirement).

- Being upset and having depression.

The treatments:

- Providing for yourself a good diet: foods having high level of iron which is found in meat, grains, tubers, vegetables and fresh fruit.

- Doing exercise frequently, walking outside, trying to breath deeply.

- Putting yourself in a cool workplace with opened windows, drinking plenty of water.

- Taking a balance between time of working and relaxing. One or two nights of deep sleeping can help you to recover quickly. During the working day, you should arrange your time to relax the muscles, take a deep breath and stop all the thinking (mental relaxation).

- Changing working habit to avoid being boring from the way you sit to the way you carry out the work in order to give yourself something new to experience.

If the phenomenon lasts more than 2 weeks, you should go to the doctor.

38. How to treat anemia

Looking in the mirror, you see a pale face with tired and lethargic state, then you may be suffering from anemia. Speaking precisely, there is a lack of red blood cells in your blood components. Red blood cells are essential for the body because they have the task of getting the oxygen in the lungs and distributing to other parts of the body.

Anemia is the iron deficiency in blood components. In the US, 20% of women at childbearing age can suffer from anemia, while only 2% of men have this disease. The reason can be that they lose a lot of blood during the menstrual period, eat a not enough amount of iron or be unable to absorb iron.

Every day our bodies must absorb 7-20mg iron when we are in pregnancy or having breastfeeding. Liver, intestine and cancer are also the possible causes of disease.

When the body loses the ability to absorb vitamin B12, it is sure that people will have anemia.

You have to find the causes to cure the disease. If the cause is only the inadequate meal, then it is lucky that you can be easily treated. Your doctor will tell you to do the following activities:

- Eating iron-rich foods: vegetables, red meat, liver, beef, chicken, ducks, birds, fish, oysters and wheat germ.

- Stimulating the ability to absorb iron by eating more fruits which are rich in vitamin C, such as citrus, tomatoes (circuit breaker) and red beet. Red meat is high in iron and have ability to stimulate the body's process of absorbing iron.

- Avoiding drinking a lot of tea, because in tea, there are substances making iron-absorbing capability slowed down.

- Drinking iron tablets after or before a meal, but no drinking iron tablets when you have an empty stomach. If doing so, the iron will make the stomach feel gnawing and uncomfortable.

39. Avoid being fainted and treatment for people getting fainted

Before fainting, you often see the darkness and everything is like doing spinning. There can be dizziness as like many stars is speckling, your face goes pale, your body generates cold sweat. Then you can fall down.

Fainting may last for several seconds or half of an hour. The cause can be that blood flow to the brain is reduced dramatically due to: emotional effect, getting tired, sudden changing positions, low sugar level in the blood, irregular heartbeat, heart attack and getting so angry.

This is what we have to do when someone get fainted:

- Advocate the victims to help them not fall down.

- Place the victim lying on the bed, so that the head is set lower than the heart and legs are propped up on high position, to ease the circulation of blood to the brain.

If the patient is placed like that, they'll still be aware of the things happening around.

- Turn the patient's head to one side, so that victim's tongue does not flow backwards inside the throat.

- Loosen the patient's clothes.

- Apply a wet cold towel on the face and the neck.

- Keep the patient warm, especially in the cold season.

Things not to do:

- Do not slap or shake the patient, especially when they are just fainted.

- Do not let the patient drink anything, even if it is water.

- Only let the patient stand up when they feel surely alright, pay attention to them during a few minutes later to make sure they are not fainted again.

If you have ever been fainted, try to find out the reason. Fainting is not a disease. Many people can be fainted together at a time in a crowd, or when they are too tired or facing something causing a huge frustration.

If you stand up suddenly and immediately feel dizzy, you may be suffering from a lower blood pressure. This situation occurs when you change positions suddenly like turning from sitting to standing up quickly. If you have already known your situation, sit down and stand up slowly, do not stand in one place for too long.

The pharmaceutical (medicines) can also make you have hypotension unexpectedly. If you notice the symptoms of dizziness after taking the medicine, ask your doctor to change medications.

Those who are often fainted should wear loose clothing to not affect the flow of blood to the small blood vessels in the end point of the circulatory system.

40. How to deal with backache

Most cases of back pain is caused by the muscles in the lower back fatigue. Simple treatments are:

- Lying on the bed with your back leaning down. Every time we move, the back will be massaged: the feeling of aches will reduce gradually. But, the time of 2-3-day lying is enough for a backache.

Lying down longer will make the muscles weaken. During convalescence, please:

- Just sit down or stand up when it is necessary. When lying, occasionally turn your body to the left and to the right, flex your feet, put hands against the bed, lift up and lay down again.

To do some exercises for the lower back, put something under the knee to relax or lying sideways with two legs bending.

The medicines are only temporary methods to relieve the pain:

- Aspirin is a drug commonly used to reduce general pain, and back pain particularly.

- Your doctor can also give you some drugs to reduce spasms of the muscles. These medicines should be taken under the guidance of doctors, including tranquilizers with codeine.

Methods of icing:

- If the pain is caused by the collision and there are broken blood vessels and muscles, you can put a towel soaked in iced water on the pain and then lay down in 20 minutes. Do so 2 to 3 times per day for 3 days.

Method of using heating pad:

- Back pain caused by torn muscle should not apply heat as this will cause more bleeding. If there is only a slight swollen spot, apply heating the pain can make the problem worse.

- You can apply heating after 4 days of icing. There are also the electric method, compressing the pain by a hot bottle or bag, using lamp to shine on the pain and hot shower. The time of treatment is often 20 minutes each time, 3 times a day.

Massaging is a good method to relieve back pain, enhance the blood flow to deliver blood to the tiny blood vessels and relax the muscles.

With strong people, they often apply waistcoat on the lower back to fix the spine and the muscles, so that they can relax.

After following the above methods, when the pain is eased, you should do exercise with gentle movements to exercise the abdomen and the lower back. At this time, you should avoid sitting for a long time. When sleeping, just lie on your back or on one side, never have a tummy state of sleeping.

After 7 days, if it is still not better, you should go to a doctor for further diagnosis, to see whether you are having these diseases:

- Kidney diseases

- Spine and spondylosis diseases

- Sciatica diseases or other related diseases.

41. How to tell a doctor about your health problem?

Mr. A has a toothache, Ms. B has broken leg, Mr. C has acne in the thigh. All these 3 people, in general, have pain, but the pain of each person is different. Therefore, when we go to a doctor to tell about our problems, the doctor always want to know the details of the situation to diagnose the disease properly.

Here are some questions your doctor may ask, if you know them in advance, we can rely on it to prepare what to tell the doctor:

- Have you ever suffered from this situation?

- When do you have pain and how frequent?

- It is a sudden pain or occasional pain?

- Whether you have pain in one place or the pain moves from one place to another?

- How long does the pain last?

- Does taking aspirin help?

- How did you do to relieve the pain? Did it get better?

- Each time you have the pain, are there any accompanying symptoms (e.g: vomiting and fatigue)?

The pain can be divided into many types with varying degrees. When telling about your pain, you should make it clear for the doctor, to find out the right treatment. You can select one of the following questions to describe the pain:

1. Mild pain

- Feeling uncomfortable

- Pain prickly

- Aching

- Dull ache

- Hurt

- Pain as being pinched

- Irritation

2. Moderate pain

- Pain to grimaces

- Pain occasionally

- Pain as beaten

- Throbbing pain

- Abdominal cramp

- Pain as being raked

- Pain that you cannot do anything.

3. Serious pain

- Pain as like your flesh was cut

- Pain as like something penetrated

- Pain as like there is stirring objects inside

- Rolling pain

- Pain to chocking

- Pain as like you have cracked skin

- Pain in tears

42. 20 questions on back pain

Back pain has many causes. Doctors need to ask the following questions to diagnose. You can also send to your doctors the answer of these questions instead of direct going to the doctor:

1. Previously, have you had back pain before?

2. Where do you feel the pain majorly? (Upper back, waist, sides, bottom)

3. When, how painful, any symptoms before the pain?

4. Instant pain or slow pain?

5. Do you have nausea, vomiting while having the pain?

6. Do you sleep well? Have you ever been awakened by the pain?

7. Is this the first time of the pain?

8. Is it a constant pain?

9. Does the pain is often interrupted?

10. Pain or dull, shallow or heavy pain?

11. Can you predict the reason? Select the following reasons:

- The weather changes

- Heavy loading

- Improper posture while standing, sitting, bending or lying

- The nerve tension

- The period

- A specific disease

- Pregnancy

- Overworking

- Other reasons

12. When do you often have the pain?

- Working

- When lifting something up

- When lying

- When bending your body

- When you have nerve tension

- When being tired

- When sewing, knitting

- When sitting

- When standing

- When driving

- When you have to carry heavy loads

- In the morning

- At noon

- In the afternoon, evening

- In other cases

13. Is the pain in one place or spread to many places?

14. Have you ever had cramping?

15. Do you lie in soft bed or hard bed?

16. Have you ever been emotionally affected or felt over-nervous?

17. Are there any red spots or swollen blisters?

18. How do you have the pain in daily life?

19. How do you often deal with the pain?

- Apply heat

- Apply cold

- Do exercise

- Have a rest

- Hot shower

- Massage, relax

- Wear waistcoat

- Walk.

20. Do you want to tell something more to your doctor?

43. Things to remember when carrying something

You just pick something up, suddenly you feel a sharp pain. If you have had back pain, you need to know the precautions.

Want to avoid the above phenomenon, when lifting something, you have to remember:

- Do not lift heavy objects.

- Bend your body higher than your waist's position to pick up something.

- Do not lift heavy objects when bending your back.

- Do not lift things while twisting the spine posture. If you want to lift it up, you just move the whole person, from head to toe, looking toward the loads.

- Do not attempt to lift an object which is above your head height.

- Do not pick up things quickly, do not jerk them upwards.

- When you lift your arms, you should distribute the loads to 2 sides of your body equally.

- Do not lift something by one hand when you are holding a baby. Put the baby down and then use two hands to lift the object.

- Need to pay attention when lifting heavy objects with high heels. You should take off shoes before lifting the object.

- When lifting something, you should stand firmly.

- Do not lift heavy objects, if you have had a backache.

When lifting, remember to:

- Wear sturdy shoes, no high heels.

- Stand in solid position, right near the objects, then lift them up.

- Bend your knees and lift things up.

- Note to use the abdominal muscles and bottom muscles to lift things

- Note to use a harmony of thighs and legs to lift the object.

- Lift things up in a position which is close to the body

- Bend your knees before lifting

- Lift slowly, if it is required, just call for help

- When you move things, try thinking about other methods instead of carrying things by yourself.

44. The pain of tennis players

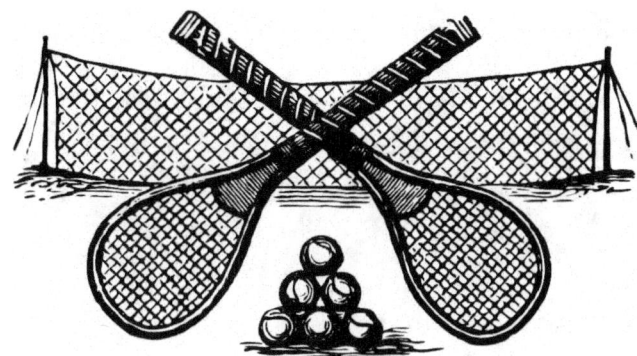

The tennis players, especially beginners, often feel pain in the elbow and the hand. There are many reasons as follows:

- Using a heavy racket

- Wire on the racket is too narrow

- Old and crushed ball

- The imbalance of the two racket's faces

- When striking, the player does not know how to use the power of the arm to coordinate with the whole body. So, the right arm overworks.

To relieve the pain, you should:

- Apply ice to the sore in the neck and elbow in 2-3 days.

- Take aspirin.

- If the pain lasts in 3 weeks, you should go to a doctor for x-ray screening or taking more medications or applying steroid injections.

- Wait for the pain to be over and then play back.

- Wear protective buckle wrist.

- Exercise the hand and the wrist by lifting light objects to slowly stretch the wrist

- Put your wrists and hands down on the table and raise your hands over your wrist while keeping being close to the table, move your hands upside down and then pick the hands up from 10 to 40 times of one turn.

45. How to deal with varicose veins

The vein in the legs is often swollen visibly under the skin and even in the knee joints, makes the patients feel hard when moving.

To prevent this problem:

- When sitting, do not cross your legs.

- Avoid standing for a long time in one place. If you have to stand when working, you should put the weight to one foot and always switch legs.

- Do not wear tight clothing to not bundle the wrist, ankles, elbows, thighs and hips.

- Eat more fruits and foods which are easily digested, constipation can easily make the blood vessels dilate.

- Always pay attention to leg movement in all positions. For example, when sitting can twist your feet, lift up your feet and legs, kick your legs forth and back, stretch your feet straight out to touch the floor, lift your legs up on the seat, etc.

A varicose vein is not dangerous. If you feel the pain in any vein, you need to ask the doctor.

46. Avoid smelly feet

Smelly feet is really unpleasant. It persists, affects the skin between the toes, especially between toes number 3 and 4. You should also know that it can spread to other people.

People who are easy to be infected are those who often go on barefoot, in the public bathroom, in the pool where there are dust, mold and fungi from others' smelly feet. Generally, people who often go to fitness clubs are easy to catch this problem, so, in America, people call this case as "athletes' foot odor"

If your feet smell, you should:

- Wash your feet at least 2 times a day, thoroughly wash and dry your toes.

- Go on shoes or sandals with open hole rather than non-airy shoes.

- If possible, change shoes every day.

Note: People with diabetes need more care for their feet to not smell, to avoid bacterial infection. People with diabetes need to keep their feet and toes airy.

47. Callosity on feet

Cause of callosity on feet is rugged spot on the foot when we wear tight shoes, the skin is harden and thicken. Do not use razor blade or sharp object to cut the callosity. Additionally, you should not take any strong chemicals to affect the callosity, because it can make the foot becomes inflamed or infected.

So, you should:

- Take the fit shoes for the foot. Do not bunch your toes.

- Soak your feet to the hot water to soften the callosity.

- Use a buffer available for sale in the stores to put under the callosity.

- If the callosity is sloughed, use a towel or a gauze soaked in 5- 10% solution of salicylic acid to cover the callosity. If the pain continues, you should go to the doctor. Many callosity go deep into the flesh as like they have roots, you must use especially curing medicine to take them out.

- If the layer of callosity is too thick, soak your feet into the hot water and then take the layer out slightly by emery. Do not cut or scratch the callosity.

People with diabetes and heart disease should pay attention to protect the nails. Be careful to prevent the callosity from turning into infection vacuum. If there are problems, go to the doctor to seek medical treatment as soon as possible, because the inflammation of the hands and feet can impact on the disease.

48. Manage the ingrown nails

Sometimes, toe nail does not grow straight. The top part of the nail, especially the curved sides can crash into the flesh, cause the swelling, pain and infection. Causes of this problem can be:

- The top part of the nail is crashed when playing sports.

- Wearing the shoes so tight.

- Cutting toenails too close. So, when the nails grow, the corner of the nail can crash into the flesh.

- Curved nails from birth.

Treatments at home:

- Soak your nails in hot water 3-4 times a day to wash your feet.

- Softly curl up the curved nail.

- Soak a cotton ball into a disinfectant solution and try to put it under your curved toenail to avoid the nail plugging in flesh.

- Repeat those 3 steps daily until the nail grows beyond pain. In these days, wear shoes to protect the sore.

If the skin is swollen with pus, you should go to the doctor, to decide whether to take antibiotics or to remove the curved nail.

As a precaution, especially for those who have had a bent nail ramming into the flesh, when cutting toenails, always cut immediately, or pay attention not to cut the top corner of the toenails too close.

Note: people with diabetes and heart disease should pay attention to protect your nails from infection.

49. The case of usual getting cold hands and feet

Many people have to wear socks all year round, even in the summer time. Their hands and feet always get cold, when the fingers are red and sometimes purple. The cause is much drug used somehow or Raynaud's disease, an ailment characterized by difficult blood circulation to the tiny blood vessels in the feet and hands. Psychosomatic diseases also cause this phenomenon. The symptoms include:

- Toes and fingers are pale, white or purple, they turn red in cold weather.

- It feels like tingling and numbness.

- Seeing the pain changing the color from red to purple or red to white.

To deal with the disease, you should:

- Stop smoking because the it slows the blood flow.

- Avoid drinking coffee because caffeine makes blood vessels narrow.

- Avoid holding cold objects. For example: do not soak hand in ice water.

- Sometimes, move your hands toward the ground, or turn two arms around in a circle, back and forth as like you are practice swimming. This action is intended to push the blood to the fingertip.

- When standing or sitting, move the fingers and feet.

- Do simple exercises to exercise the muscles (see section number 160 'Stress treatment').

Chapter 2: Some things to note about disease prevention, diagnostic and treatment

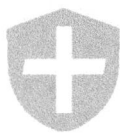

We should be most worried about what? Work, spending or health?

If I had to choose one of three answers above, you have chosen to make the first sentence 3. Since an infected person cannot maintain employment but must spend mutilated.

Early disease detection is important: good support poor and shorten the healing time, sometimes even save lives because treated promptly.

This chapter serves as a map to help you find out the path to follow in order to tackle difficulties related to health.

50. Alzheimer's disease of old age

We haven't yet to find out the cause of illness, just know that the disease usually get acquainted with people over 80 years old. Few people under 65 years of age with this disease. Is it because a certain virus or not? It remains a question, on the way to find the culprit weaken - sometimes destructive - the brain cells responsible for receiving, storing and processing information.

Alzheimer's disease symptoms include:

- The ability to pay attention is reduced.

- Performance of the bowel and bladder weakness sometimes, losing control.

- Physical Impairment.

- Disorientation

- Forgetfulness (usually new things happen).

- Become clumsy.

- Say no clear, coherent.

- Or sorrow, anger.

- Confusing.

- Or miss the daily work.

There are also patients with Alzheimer's disease-like symptoms such as brain tumors, cerebral hematoma, a lack of vitamin B12, thyroid depression. These diseases are treatable. Since there are no medicines Alzheiner, so if a family history of the disease should do some of the following to help patients perform daily tasks:

Making a loud reminder letters stating what to do during the day.

- Technical Advice patients treated sequentially table and the

- For the capital used in place provisions to the patient catchy and accessible place.

- Technical Advice or write to a table when things are done to remind something. For example: the "closing memory", "water course" near the faucet, etc.

- Always pay attention to the patient's meal with all the necessary nutrients.

- Creating conditions for the patient and a walk with the family.

Create air to see his patients remain an active part of the family.

51. Distinguish angina and heart attack

Chest pain often has symptoms such as:

- Chest pain, you feel like there is any heavy object on the chest

- Feeling like chest bumps

- The pain spreads from the chest to the arms and neck

- Hands feel heavy, tremors and numbness difficult to move (usually the right)

- The discomfort, bloating fatigue as being.

Someone has a heart attack after suffering chest pain, but the fact the two conditions are different. Only those who already have heart disease, the new chest pain is a heart attack harbinger of the future.

However, it is easy to confuse the two diseases together because they have a similar number of reasons such as:

- The pain occurs when the heart vessels with fat embolism suspensions or slow blood flow to the heart

- In both cases, the patients were seen spreading from chest pain to the arms, shoulders and neck (pain from a heart attack usually 30 minutes long, while the pain of chest pain from just a few seconds longer to Few minute).

- Both cases occur when the patient is doing something heavy requires more effort.

- Often happens to men over 50 and women after menopause.

Doctors often ask patients to differentiate the two diseases and are often based on the following considerations:

- After a heart attack, the patient is still feeling pain because the heart muscle is damaged. Chest pain who often do not see that.

- The pains were cardiac chest pain anemia, but often just take a break to recover health is seen immediately. Whether people are resting heart but still feel tired, long recovery ..

- Use nitroglycerine, chest pain who find effective immediately. But for a heart attack, this medication has no effect.

Yet doctors still have to conduct some further tests before concluding the pain of the type of disease (eg ECG).

In addition, the following factors can lead to chest pain.

- Recently a meal too, are more difficult to digest.

- Just being one "shock" because a sad or happy, surprise.

- Have high blood pressure.

- The rate of high blood cholesterol than normal levels allow.

- Smoking.

- A family history of heart attack (chest pain genetics). If you often have chest pain, should:

- See your doctor for instructions on using nitroglycerine or effective drugs dilating the coronary arteries to ease blood flow to the heart. Nitroglycerine medications such effects when taking 1 to 2 minutes.

- Must quit smoking because the nicotine in tobacco makes the blood vessels narrower.

- Avoid foods difficult to digest.

- After eating, take a break or do light work.

- Restricting out when windy, cold.

- Limit fat intake to lower the rate of cholesterol.

- Avoid any situation that makes me angry to worry, touching.

52. Arthritis

When the cartilage in joints is damaged or infected with certain causes, people will feel pain in the joints, every move, it was arthritis. If inflamed because of infection, need to consult a doctor to receive treatment as soon as possible. Symptoms of arthritis include:

- Feel the limbs, stiff.

- Some joints swollen.

- Joint pain, aching inside.

- Every time you move back pain.

- Joints stiff and red.

- Fever, weight loss, fatigue.

There are many types of arthritis, but notable 3 common types:

1. Arthritis of the elderly due to cartilage compression and friction over the years, worn for her age. Elderly often feel sore and stiff limbs in the afternoon.

2. Rheumatic disease characterized by swollen at the toes, fingers, wrists, feet, elbows, knees, causing stiffness in the morning, about an hour long. Women aged 30 - 40 or more men.

3. Frequently spondylitis disease in men aged 15 to 45 years is characterized by pain at the end of the spine for back pain accompanying phenomenon.

Normally doctors often treated as follows:

- Give aspirin painkillers and anti-inflammatory drug (no drug-steroidal type).

- Bed rest, warm compresses or ice only.

- A set of exercises suitable for diseases, related to the painful area to enhance the motility of joints.

Exercise is the best means discovered all measures have the effect of limbs easily stretch to withstand the weight, tension, strengthen the contraction of muscles and so on ...

However, the training needs to be doctors instructions, for practicing too hard will cause more pain.

Swimming is a good form of exercise because the pool of body weight was water-lifting, longer legs, arms and all joints in the body are gentle agitation.

Generally, exercise should treat attention.

- Select the appropriate exercises to mobilize the joints pain.

- Set slow slightly and then slowly increase the intensity.

- If there is no pain because the practice match, they must stop practicing painful movements.

- Do not overdo. Tap done to have time off commensurate with the fatigue of training hard.

- To focus attention on the effective movement to the joints, especially when campaigning in the country.

- Train to persist.

53. Take early detection of cancer

It is assumed that in the US, the number of deaths due to cancer ranks 2nd, after a number of deaths due to heart disease. Often up to 30% of the US population potentially infected, most cases of lung cancer, colon, rectum, breast, bladder, prostate and uterus.

Fortunately, the cancer figures are not greater than 70%. However, each person must pay attention on how to keep yourself standing in that 70% figure. For this, we must:

- No smoking.

- Eat light, easily digested.

- Drink little or no alcohol.

- Maintain a clean environment. Avoid breathing polluted air for chemicals.

- Avoid sun much.

To note comments and detect changes or abnormalities on their base to report immediately to your doctor. The early detection brings much hope could save the lives of myself. These abnormalities are:

- The operation is not normal bladder, the bowel.

- There lymph node or lump in the breast or anywhere else.

- Bleeding though not unusual menstrual periods, or prolonged menstruation (women) in the anus (male and female).

- Hoarseness or pertussis no cure.

- Sore throat not long off.

- There are changes in the strange wart, mole.

- Swallowing hard and dyspepsia, prolonged.

54. Cataracts

Patients find themselves standing in a layer of haze. Even in broad daylight, but everything around them blurred. Evening, worse. Sometimes, looking at a reification two, light as eye pain: it is teased stock of cataracts.

Previously, it was thought that the disease of the elderly. But not! Causes disease is caused by too much exposure to ultraviolet rays. Therefore, take sun hat, hat, wear eye protection is good and necessary method to not develop cataracts later.

Some other symptoms of this disease are:

- Do not recognize the colors.

- Or was blinding, especially in the evening.

Glasses for near vision (old glass), are no longer effective. A large number of patients with this disease are often beyond the age of 40 and had surgery to treat. 97% of surgeries have obtained good results. However, the need to have surgery or not, should be left to doctors to decide.

Previously, after the surgery, the patient must wear thick glasses the eyes to adjust. Now, doctors can be attached directly to the small lenses in the eye pupil is very convenient for users.

After eye surgery, patients still have to pay attention to avoid ultraviolet rays. Whenever the sun, should wear sunglasses.

55. Chronic power Syndrome

Over ten years ago, from the early '80s, many American medical research focused on a disease that impair the health of women aged 20 to 40 years old. Men are also, but less. Most of them are intellectuals, have a stable professional career. Symptoms of this disease are. People get tired, feel strength gradually decline, accompanied by at least 6 months:

- Sore throat.

- Swollen

- Mild fever, a headache, dizziness.

- The moody.

- Sore muscles.

- Weight loss.

- Memory decline.

Patients always feel like I was seasick on a boat or floating in the waves. The symptoms that make professionals think about diseases like AIDS, tuberculosis, mental etc ..., but the tests did not find the bacteria or virus. So far, the cause of the disease remains shrouded in secrecy. The doctors only agreed to get together about naming the disease is "chronic human syndrome", they named the virus may be the culprit causing this disease is Epstein Barr and advise the patient should:

- Rest, convalescence.

- Read the documentation to know how to avoid stress and nervous diseases stress.

- Know how to monitor their health.

- Healthy living.

- Contact with sick people like me to learn from experience.

56. Cirrhosis

The liver of the body keeps a lot of functions in our body:

- Production of honey to participate in the digestion of fat.

- Production of proteins in the blood.

- Create a clotting agent.

- Cholesterol Metabolism.

- Keep a reasonable rate of sugar in the blood components.

- As of glycogen storage reserves.

- Participating in the production of more than 1,000 kinds of enzymes have different effects in the body.

- Filter and remove the harmful toxins in the body, such as alcohol and pharmaceutical.

The liver can tolerate a certain amount of alcohol. But if people drink alcohol always, drink plenty of the damaged liver. The residual fat in the liver closed, destroy the liver causing cirrhosis, common in men over 45 years old. The number of American women with cirrhosis before less, now also increase.

People who drink often do not eat enough because more and more they should drink more than the body missing vitamins and minerals you need.

Cirrhosis bile duct leading to pain and jaundice. The oral drug to treat liver to make more tired. Doctors often based on the following symptoms to conclude patients with cirrhosis:

- Enlarged liver.

- Long eyes are yellow and white.

- Urine brown (the color of tea).

- Classification can be bloody.

- Hair loss.

- Consistent legs and swollen stomach (tripe).

- Weakness nervous.

Fatal cirrhosis. The treatment takes a long time so it is better not to drink!

57. Sick myocardial infarction

Every day, 4,000 Americans have heart attacks, muscle pain in each time reachs to about 20 seconds. Each year about 600,000 people die of myocardial infarction related to coronary artery. Heart disease has the highest number of victims compared to other diseases in the United States. Fortunate that in recent years, the number of deaths from the disease tends to be reduced because of the conditions a few good eating, exercise movements, medicine pushed enough and most of them are about disease.

Organization of American cardiovascular disease prevention recommend that people should:

- Regularly check your blood pressure. High blood pressure will facilitate the scaling of fat in blood vessels, among them the coronary arteries. The cardiovascular specialist will give you further instructions about diet should follow (do not eat much salt to control the amount of sodium in the blood. It should pay attention to weight, because overweight also affects blood pressure TOP, causing high blood pressure ...).

- Quit smoking because nicotine causes vasoconstriction as blood flow to the heart and less, do not provide enough oxygen to the heart. It also said that nicotine can directly affect the heart and coronary arteries.

- Ask your doctor to check for diabetes related diseases through to coronary heart disease.

- Keep the weight just right. Obese people too vulnerable to high blood pressure, diabetes, heart attack than other people.

- There are limited dietary fat and cholesterol with foods such as lean meats, vegetables, vegetable oil. These foods have a high proportion of fat and cholesterol fats facilitate scaling as congested blood vessels, including arteries in the heart.

- Aerobic exercise at least 3 times a week, every 20 minutes. Sitting work day after day, every month, every year will lead to heart disease later on (see Chapter 3 for the benefit of the subjects go, running, cycling).

- Implement methods stretchy self-training to have grand visions about things happening around us every day. The neurological disease, stress related phenomenon intimately phenomenon of high blood pressure and heart disease - arteries.

- Take regular check on Tim - circuit. You need to know the symptoms of heart disease - at the circuit to occur, go immediately to a place of cure, do not leave until it's too late.

Here are the symptoms of the disease myocardial infarction:

- Seeing discomfort or chest pain lasts for several minutes.

- The feeling of discomfort or pain, spreading to the shoulders, neck, hands and jaws.

- Feeling nausea, vomiting or nausea and vomiting along with chest pain.

- Cold sweats.

- Shortness of breath.

- Dizziness, vertigo.

- Belly hangover (stomach rumbling).

- Feeling worried, as predictable upcoming disaster.

If you knew you had a heart attack (myocardial infarction - coronary artery obstruction ...) go to the hospital or emergency room immediately!

Quick is expected to survive. Is likely to die slowly.

58. Colitis

The last part of the small intestine, large intestine is connected to the right side of the abdomen, of us. When this period is inflamed, we see the following symptoms:

- Pain in the lower abdomen, right side. Often pain after meals.

- Diarrhea (no blood).

- A slight fever.

- Nausea, vomiting.

- Loss of appetite, weight loss.

- Pain, inflammation of the anus.

- Joint pain.

- Tired.

They call this disease is Crohn's disease, more common in patients aged 15 to 35 years old in Europe, the South Caucasus and the Jewish people. The disease appears as a plague, come and go, do not know the cause so unpredictable. The medication is a cure diarrhea, inflammatory treatment (antibiotics), vitamins and sometimes aided composition steroid drugs.

During abdominal illness should apply heat to relieve pain, drink plenty of water to compensate for the loss of water, rest. 70% of patients often require surgery because the disease may spread outside the junction between the small intestine and colon.

Avoid eating milk, eggs, flour and other foods that are high in fiber. Because inflammation may develop more seats.

Avoid drinking alcohol.

Eat vitamin-rich substances, proteins and carbohydrates. Patients should be treated because doctors can complication of other intestinal diseases.

59. Diabetes

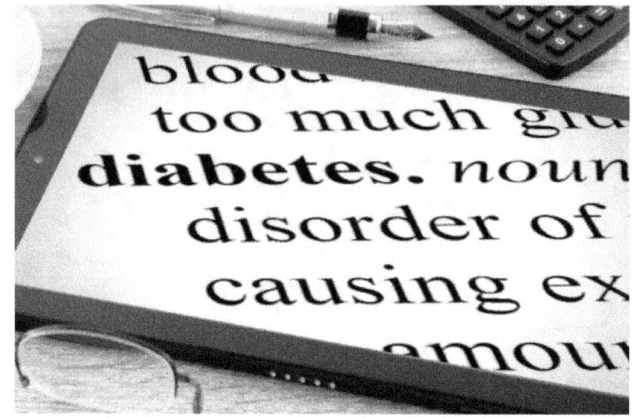

The system of our body is responsible for transformation of sugar into glucose for the body like "ét chancre" for motorcycles so.

When insulin - a hormone secreted by the pancreas, a lack of glucose in the blood increases incompatible with the normal rate of substances in the blood. The kidneys filter blood to remove glucose excreted in the urine: it is diabetes.

The cause of the disease is caused by insulin deficiency, the doctor injured patients taking injections or insulin medications. The symptoms of diabetes include:

- Sleepiness, drowsy.

- Itching.

- Blurred vision.

- Heavy movement.

- Tinnitus, hands, feet cold, pain.

- Ease tired.

- Skin infections easier, cuts hands, feet, scrapes - especially in the legs - healing.

- A family history of diabetes.

People with diabetes often frequent urination (going always) always thirsty and hungry, fast weight loss, fatigue or irritability, or voice-headed and nauseous, vomiting.

No need to have all of these symptoms are sick. If a family member who already have the disease, then you have a blood test every year, at least once in the year because of this genetic disease.

There are 2 types of diabetes:

1. Heavy type, including people under 40 also suffer. When required insulin treatment.

2. lighter type common in the elderly and obese. For these patients, sometimes just eating under special regime from, such as dietary fat, eating less or fasting sugar, eat more fibrous substances v. v ...

Exercise is good for patients because apparently the movements of the body can affect the regulation of insulin. Therefore, the body does not keep a meaty, with careful diet, exercise capacity is 3 effective remedies to prevent diabetes.

60. Inflammatory bowel wall

Human intestinal wall is not straight smooth peaks and troughs that are slightly both inside and outside. If inside the concave depressions too will like these small bags, waste accumulation of digestive apparatus on the road formed to expel the stool. That is the point of causing inflammation, intestinal cramps and pain in the lower abdomen, the left side.

The creation of small sacs disadvantages such as a malformation of the intestine unfortunately. We are not curable but can be prevented by:

- Note to eat more foods high in fiber, fresh vegetables, bread made from grain starch.

- Avoid eating the bread, jam with small particles (guava, pomegranate) because the particles are easily trapped in the pocket in the process of digestion.

The intestinal pain symptoms include:

- Analysis of blood.

- A slight fever, the chills.

- Lower abdominal pain every time when intestines or tummy tuck operation.

61. Shortness of breath emphysema

Certification emphysema or dyspnea is a lung disease. Patients who have always felt the lack of air around them, like breathing in the first situation was taken in a plastic bag so. America has a million people like that. Their follicles damaged lungs, so 2 lungs lose elasticity to stretch out and bend when inhaled while breathing emissions. In short, their lungs are not done well the movements of respiration.

There are 3 to 5 percent of people infected in areas where hazardous substances contaminate the environment. And the majority, over 50% of those over 50 years old, addicted to cigarettes. Therefore, it is also called dyspnea or emphysema is a disease of smokers.

Shortness of breath develop into disease over a long period. Many patients do not show symptoms of severe illness before. The symptoms may be as follows:

- Cough, with profuse.

- Breathe through your mouth.

- Shortness of breath, a wheezing.

- Ease tired.

- The thin, clear bone, rapid weight loss.

Doctors usually test more to clear the disease by means of X-rays. sputum, lung and ask about family history to see if anyone was not working. When concluded patients suffering from emphysema, there were 50-70% of lung tissue was destroyed, the doctor will ask the patient:

- Try to plan to quit smoking.

- Avoid areas where smoke and polluted environment.

- Take measures to reduce mucus in the lungs.

- Daily exercise.

- There are enough quality dietary allowances.

- Drink lung drugs, drugs with steroids and antibiotics.

- Injecting drugs and medicines against tuberculosis flu annually.

Emphysema long and hard to cure fully recovered should question and avoid disease prevention first.

62. Gallstone disease

If you encounter a person familiar with the face's hip hup obese people, please do not think they are healthy hurry. If they or bloating, especially after meals that are high in fat sometimes pain in the upper abdomen for hours, to the right, then tell them to pay attention, so maybe they were gallstone disease.

Usually there are 16 million Americans suffer from this disease, the majority are women. A few feel the symptoms. The majority saw nothing. Painful gallstone disease and require surgery to remove the stones. It is not clear already formed stones like, for whatever reason. But the forecast is due to the excess cholesterol in the blood - the same cause of cardiovascular disease.

Some people are more susceptible to gallstone disease because:

- Genetic. In families who have gallstone disease.

- Fat.

- Already in middle age and older (40 -50).

- Women in pregnancy.

- Has estrogen pills (supplements ovaries).

- Having diabetes.

- Eat lots of fat and high cholesterol foods.

- Sick of the small intestine.

To treat the disease, doctors often fed drugs to gravel, ultrasound methods used to melt the stones, remove the stone surgery, special dietary requirements less fat to avoid further large gravel.

Therefore, people who have the disease should:

- Eat foods that are high in fiber, fresh fruits and vegetables.

- Eat less or fasting fat, especially animal fat

- Avoid foods that are high in sugar.

63. Glaucoma

Glaucoma is a disease with hereditary diseases should be a highly visible 20 ~ 20 can also someday, with this disease. Once infected, the optic nerve is damaged gradually, up to the blind. If treated well, visibility is impaired.

We should know some about this disease:

- The disease is caused by the increased pressure of the fluid inside the eyeball - sometimes occurs rapidly - causing soreness and redness; require surgery to treat.

- Many patients do not notice any symptoms prior notice. In addition to the phenomenon seen blurred vision or seeing the green ring, red ... colorful when looking at a bright spot.

- The disease can be exacerbated if taking certain medications or anti-histamine type of anti-muscle contraction.

To prevent glaucoma, which can lead to blindness, when the phenomenon of suspicion of the disease, have to treat eye specialist immediately. Your doctor will give you medication or special treatment using eye drops to reduce intraocular pressure (eye pressure when rising, see eye pain).

In addition, we also use these methods:

- Ultrasound to reduce intraocular pressure.

- Laser surgery fast, remove some fluid in the eyeball out.

64. Gout (hands, feet, joints)

If you suddenly woke up at midnight and saw the big toe pain, so, you can be gout. Along with the thumb can hurt both the instep, heel, foot wrist, elbow, knee. The bridles just slight friction with sharp pain bed supply. Furthermore you can see people chills and mild fever. Gout is an arthritis-like disease species, common in men over 50, there is protein in the body is reduced leading to increased uric acid in mau.Chat of uric acid can crystallize and the crystals as the smell of needles into the tendons in the joints, causing swelling and intense pain. They also can have such effects in the kidney and in the subcutaneous adipose tissue. The pain can last from a few hours to a few days, after the patient:

- Being injured or vessels collided in the joints.

- Drink.

- Eat more red meat such as liver, kidneys, tongue ...

- Eat sardines and anchovies.

- Taking diuretic drugs.

When hurt, you should to visit hospital for the doctor only new assertiveness is it true that you do not gout. There are a number of other diseases have similar symptoms of gout. The doctor also must be tested to see if excess uric acid is excreted by the body too much or weak kidneys do not work fully discharged.

For treatment, the doctor will think of ways to reduce the pain, and then find ways to reduce the amount of acid in the blood by UNC Oral anti-inflammatory medications and avoiding the movements required to not touch the pain bridles.

- Stop drinking, drink plenty of water

- Limit your intake of meat, especially red meat.

65. High blood pressure

Unlike diseases such as toothache, a headache, constipation, etc., a person with high blood pressure cannot feel anything unusual at all. So, they can be easily killed. Therefore, one room for high blood pressure are: Hungarian Prime Quiet name. Each year, this disease has to over one million Americans. 95% of them do not know they are sick, whether he wanted to know if you have high blood pressure or not? So easy!

You go your blood pressure at every opportunity and should measure always convenient. If you find yourself high blood pressure, do not worry because the waist can quickly have many causes: worry or strong emotions, drink more than- coffee, eat a lot of meat ... All of these things can make blood your pressure rise, but not for long. If after several attempts measurements and tests, doctors concluded with high blood pressure, you should follow the instructions of him as:

- Let her go weight (if overweight).

- No smoking.

- Limit alcohol.

- Limit salt intake.

- Exercise at least 3 times per week.

- Learn to relax your body and nervous to avoid stress

- Take the medication as directed by your doctor. Do not give up or intermittent drinking, though felt he had seemed normal then.

- If you are a woman, talk to your doctor about the medications you are taking contraceptives. If there is no impact to patient medication must be changed other contraceptive methods.

- Avoid using the component drugs phenyl - propanolamine.

People often measure blood pressure using an instrument consisting of two main parts: the parts wrapped in the upper arm and clock measurements.

Measurements at the clock said index by mmHg blood pressure. The first figure - high - said the biggest pressure on the blood vessels when the heart beats and contraction (systolic number).

The second number - a low number - said the pressure of blood on arteries when the heart expands (diastolic). Results comparing two numbers of systolic / diastolic for people to assess the current status of how your blood pressure. For example, normal blood pressure is 120/80.

The following is a record of the assessment body's blood pressure, applies to adults aged 18 and older. To evaluate properly, so measured repeatedly at different times, and each time, scoring from 2 to many of systolic / diastolic. Thidu: 90 or higher diastolic blood pressure that is worse than both the systolic is 160.

66. Kidney stones

Between deep sleep, John suddenly woke up. He felt a sharp pain in the lower abdomen sides. Three years ago, he had once been like that, and the doctor has ordered him to the laboratory. The results showed that urinary calcium and John have more uric acid: His kidneys have a small gravel particles. Back then, doctors were treating him with hot water immersion method: John is sitting on a special chair placed in a tub of hot water flooding to the neck. They create and control the waves for wave hitting pebbles kidney area making in breaking into pieces. Then, he had plenty of water to waste scrap pieces of gravel that out through the urine.

Kidney stones often go, is back. Sick people, should follow the following instructions:

- When urinating pebbles, gravel should seize, put to the test your doctor and work out the appropriate treatment plan. Follow your doctor's advice if kidney stones created by calcium, patients must not eat foods high in calcium too. If the stone is formed by uric acid, patients should limit their consumption of protein-rich food, and drinking alkaline bicarbonate to reduce the sodium tri substances in the body. Drink plenty of water daily, intermittent 2 liters / day. Go to medical examination the doctor periodically to monitor the functioning of the kidneys.

67. Lung cancer

Now think back, when people were found unknown of cigarettes and the air is less polluted, then lung cancer is a strange disease, less noticeable. And now, every year up to 150,000 Americans, both men and women, they have this disease, 85%

of them were smokers. Worse yet, the number of female patients is increasing. The number of women dying from lung cancer is to run a race with the number of deaths from breast cancer! The reason lung cancer is often fatal because it spreads very rapidly by the system of blood vessels carry oxygen from the lungs throughout the body away. When identified a patient with lung cancer, the other organs in the body they are infected already.

These symptoms include:

- Chronic Cough;

- Bloody sputum;

- Shortness of breath, wheezing;

- Chest pain;

- Weight loss;

- Tired.

Based on the type of illness and disease duration, the doctor will do surgery to remove part of the lung cancer, then to treatment with X-rays, or chemical. Curing cancer is difficult to do, but preventative is easy to implement: no smoking! The specialist has found that a smoker how much more likely to develop lung cancer is increasing much.

68. Sick sclerosis nerve sheaths (MS)

If our brain is like a telephone, the nerves throughout the body's network of receiving and transporting information to anywhere. Just part of the cord sheath is damaged is the acquisition of information is no longer accurate, would be weakened or broken. The nerve fibers are very fragile man, also wrapped outside by a protective membrane. When sclerosis, this protective film can swell and decompose leaving scars on the horizontal and vertical pinched nerve fibers. This phenomenon can occur in the spinal cord and brain. Usually when active, the nerve impulses travel at the speed stretch 365km / h. phenomenon in the membrane stiffness, the ability to transmit impulses are weakened, or lost. People with this disease, see:

- Lost apparent power, the weakening.

- Legs, hands, who, paralyzed;

- It is difficult to coordinate the movements;

- Bladder (bladder) perform poorly;

- May be blurred or blind in one eye.

It is not clear the cause of the disease, only commented that:

- Patients often intermittent aged 20-40.

- There may be a family member has had the disease (genetics).

- Women suffer more than men (3 vs. 2 men and women).

- In the northern United States, Canada and northern Europe many people with this disease. Because no effective treatment measures, should advise patients:

- Rest convalescence;

- Try to avoid making her nervous fatigue, avoid stress;

- Avoid hot baths. Better cold shower;

- Try to complete self-service tasks daily;

- Take exercise;

- Practice the massage to maintain the operation of the facility;

- There should be caregivers, counseling;

- You can take medication or cortisone muscle relaxation.

69. Parkinson's disease (paralysis and trembling hands)

When Louise saw her husband on the shakes hands forever, she took him to the hospital. The doctor told her, her husband with Parkinson's disease, a disease that paralyzed and trembling hands. People with Parkinson's disease also have these symptoms:

- Rigid movement, slowly.

- Let go step by step, every step to stop.

- The voice steady.

- At nap.

- Surface dull.

- Difficult to regulate postures: standing, sitting ...

- Crazy.

It is not yet know the cause, but have tried many cures, hope to help more than a million Americans - a large number of the elderly - better.

The commonly used drugs such as bromocriptine, have the effect of increasing the amount of dopamine in the brain. (Dopamine is a substance essential for the activity of the nerve cells); warm bath for patients to do the muscles are soft. Patient care, should:

- Store items can be dangerous for patients: knives, scissors ...

- Simple tasks for easy patient (eg, instead tying his shoes with slip on shoes is going to be).

- For patients eat more foods with fiber and drink plenty of water.

- Always motivate, encourage patients to patient activity.

- He should have professional care.

70. Sick stomach ulcers and duodenal

Gastric ulcer and duodenal ulcer (part of small intestine) are 2 of the digestive system diseases, common in middle-aged patients at intervals, in both men and women. After eating about an hour and a half to three hours, they often feel pain right above the navel. The pain may make sleeping person wakes up. Eat a piece of bread or drinking water reduces acidity, can support several minutes of pain.

It is unclear the cause would only be guessed by excess stomach acid and protects the tissue inside the stomach or duodenum were scrapes. Who has suffered back pain often goes painful. The next time interval from the last 2 years. People with stomach ulcers or duodenal ulcers often have symptoms:

- Pain in waves. Each session lasts from a few days of pain coming months.

- When pain is seen as bloating, pain in the heart, and feel hungry.

- Nausea and vomiting.

- Loss of appetite and weight loss.

To determine a patient with stomach pain or pain doctors duodenum based on the X-ray examination or endoscopy (colonoscopy is a method of optical instruments inserted through the patient's mouth into the stomach to look see internal state through the screen).

Here are the instructions, the patient. Should follow:

- Eat light, eat as many meals, avoid eating it.

- Avoid stimulants, including coffee, tea, soft drinks, coffee drinks - coffee.

- Avoid taking medicines affecting as aspirin ulcer ...

- Do not smoke. The number of people smoking and gastric ulcers are more than the number of people smoking.

- Try to autonomy, to avoid his being nervous tension and tress. These phenomena have the effect of additional diseases.

71. Phlebitis

The press had a top time in the news about President Richard Nixon suffered severe phlebitis. Characteristics of the disease is a blood clot phenomenon in a vein, usually in the legs. This lady or illness than men. It distinguishes between two categories:

- Inflammation of superficial veins, located just under the skin. People with varicose veins are very susceptible to this disease. Vein inflammation usually redness, palpable hard and hot. Still can heal yourself at home.

- Deep vein inflammation need to stay in hospital for treatment. Your doctor may have blood-thinning drugs to prevent the formation of another clot. When the blood clot breaks, small parts that can cause vascular congestion in the arms, legs. If this phenomenon occurs in the heart, the lungs, can cause death.

Phlebitis disease only a symptom: pain in the arms, legs. However, half of the patients with deep vein inflammation did not show any symptoms. The disease usually occurs after a period of lying convalescence after surgery, pregnancy, or taking birth control pills.

Those susceptible phlebitis are:

- The campaign refused a job or a long leisurely bored; to sit in place as long as there is occupation going ships, aircraft.

- Smoking or chewing tobacco;

- Overweight;

- Being a foot injury as bumps or falls;

- Being infected by injecting the blood vessels;

- Have some malignant diseases;

- Old Age.

Only a doctor can distinguish two kinds of phlebitis mentioned above. If you have shallow phlebitis, surely you will be doctors recommend as follows:

- For sore feet a break, not advocacy. When located, high footrest attention on the heart level until disease remission.

- Apply warm water on the pain many times during the day. Each time about 20 minutes long.

- Taking aspirin to reduce pain or type of nonsteroidal anti-inflammatory drugs such as ibuprofen.

- Avoid bedridden.

To avoid deep vein inflammation, should:

- Avoid prolonged standing or sitting for too long.

- Avoid taking oral contraceptives.

- When sitting, do not cross-legged milking (cross-legged)

- Avoid carrying things tied legs buckle as making it hard for blood to flow.

- You can lie in bed set in the case must lie down as follows: clamp a pillow between your feet. Imagine the pillow like a ball, using a leg press down to the ball deflated and then raised his foot. Went back and forth several times, then switch legs.

72. Pneumonia

Pneumonia can be treated with antibiotics. Yet, some people die from this disease still ranks 6th among the victims died from the disease in the United States. The disease develops when the lungs are infected with bacteria - virus, fungi or toxins that cause inflammation, irritation. Across the world, this nation can have more pneumonia and other ethnic groups. The disease usually attacks:

- Elderly: as people become older, the resistance of the body against disease decreases.

- People in the hospital (because of illness or occupational)

- People with a cough after a fight or beaten.

- People who smoke tobacco because tobacco paralyze hair cells tasked push the mucus out of the lungs.

- People who are malnourished (food shortage), alcoholism or was ill because the virus.

- Persons who have chronic lung disease, and emphysema.

- People with anemia.

- People with cancer are treated with X-rays or chemicals. To cure the results, should:

- Well take a long time to convalescence.

- Use the air conditioner for proper humidifier in the bedroom or any room patients often stay longer in the day.

- Drink a lot of water.

- Use adequate doses of the drug has been appointed doctor.

- Do not look at them, especially when the feeling needs to cough expectorant.

73. Reye Syndrome

Parents will want to have some knowledge of medicine to cope with situations when children are sick, poisoning, bleeding or fever. Therefore, the need to clarify more about Reye's syndrome, a disease that attacks the brain and the patient's liver, sometimes leading to death.

It is not known exactly what causes the disease, only the symptoms of the disease such as swelling of the liver and liver of the patient brain enlarged because increased fat, loss of the ability to perceive the metal elements. This causes the brain to swell and pressure of the fluid around the brain increases.

Reye's syndrome usually occurs when the patient has a lung disease related to the flu, chickenpox. These are good conditions for developing Reye syndrome and the symptoms:

- Vomiting ;.

- Dizziness;

- Easy to anger, struggle;

- Very tired, possibly coma;

- Syncope and may die.

If you suspect a child is sick, take her to the emergency room immediately. The doctor will use all methods to support brain swelling.

It is said that the use of aspirin to treat chickenpox or the flu in patients from 19 years and under, can lead to Reye's syndrome. Thus, for younger patients, or no drug, or acetaminophen instead of aspirin.

74. Scoliosis

Scoliosis usually occurs with children from 10 to 15 years old. Some of the girls are more than 7- 9 times more than the son. It is still unknown causes. The disease does not cause pain and developed slowly as the top of the crooked spine, shoulder blade on one side while the other curved hanging down are affecting both the chest and spine, as patients sometimes have to bend people out front while going or standing.

Adults with this disease is due to childhood diseases. This incurable disease doctors monitor patients only to have precautions against heart disease and lung might happen next.

The measures may apply to the patient, including:

- Give the person wearing clothes sewn especially appropriate for each patient to bending, straightening a portion of the bone, the bone in the process of development.

- For electric at some point in the spine, contributing to shaping the bone.

- If excessive crooked spine, sometimes surgery and how to re-create the spine by leaning against a piece of metal wire.

However, people still try to treat young children to prevent children from getting the disease complications later, when the children grow up.

75. The lack of red blood cells sickle Stock

One in 12 black Americans carriers the germ of deficiency to sickle red blood cells, and is capable of producing a child with this disease. If both spouses are ill 2, the number of children with genetic diseases is 25% under - 1 out of 4 children, have the disease.

Lack of sickle red blood cells, carries oxygen to every function in the body cells of the blood is impaired. The disease has no symptoms until the child turns 1. From 2 to 5 years old, the disease appear at any time and can lead to death. Blood tests, one can detect the disease. In addition, there are the following symptoms:

- Seeing the pain of mild to severe pain in the chest, joints, back or abdomen;

- Hand, foot swell;

- Yellow skin;

- Often sick, repetitive, especially pneumonia and brain membrane pain;

- Kidney failure;

- Have bladder stones (at advanced age);

- Ease of fainting (at advanced age),

It is not a curable disease, only measures to avoid complications can occur such as:

- Duration of pain, pain medications may be used, or compresses soaked in water, give oxygen.

- Injecting drug pneumonia prevention.

- The couple must take a blood test to know who has the disease gene to avoid giving birth with germs.

When a woman becomes pregnant, may be tested by means of amniocentesis for the sick or pregnant and decide whether to keep the pregnancy or not.

76. Certificate stroke

Ted is a good tennis player. Yet for some time now, he suddenly found his arms unusually weak and decided to ask the doctor. Examination and testing indicate: blood flow to the brain is not enough because the carotid artery (in the neck arteries carrying blood to the brain) may be narrowed by atherosclerosis. This phenomenon can cause syncope, fainting. To treat, Ted had to undergo a minor surgery.

Witness fainted be considered a disease involving the brain, with the death toll ranks 3rd in the US.

Brain caused by ischemia, also means lack of oxygen due to carotid artery stenosis or stroke.

Both cases are made 2 injured brain to fatal levels. To prevent disease, should:

- Check your blood pressure regularly. If necessary, take medication by a doctor appointed. Drinking a steady and sufficient dose; To reduce blood cholesterol levels less than 200 mg / dl (milligrams / deciliter);

- Exercise regularly;

- Keep non-fat too. If overweight, weight loss must seek to do;

- No smoking;

- If you have diabetes, keep your blood sugar levels should not be higher than allowed levels;

- If necessary, to stop taking birth control pills to switch to another contraceptive method. If oral contraceptives, not smoking;

- Learn methods to avoid stress.

The feel or know the warning signs of stroke certification is very important. Take the victim to the emergency where time will eliminate the harmful effects. The symptoms of fainting include :.

- Dizziness, vertigo.

- Temporary memory loss, inability to discern.

- Legs, hands, face, cold, people fall apart, weakness.

- Speaking stuttered or not speak.

- Temporary visual loss (not seen during symptomatic patients) or see Figure 2 (see 1 of 2)

- Recently an intense headache.

Some people get a slight fainting spells as warning symptoms of a more serious attack coming fainted. Because knew that, so after fainting the first time, they have time to consult a doctor to prevent fainting episodes later.

77. The malfunction of the thyroid gland

Thyroid is one of the endocrine glands, have an important role to the entire human body. Thyroid small butterfly shaped like two in front of trachea, function 2 hormones secrete thyroxine and L-thyronine L-. Two hormones that affect the progression of the phenomenon thousands metabolism in the body. When the thyroid gland is not normal activity, the hormone is produced is not strictly required by the body to make the body is disturbed. There are two cases:

Where the excess hormone (hyperthyroidism), causing the stock:

- Run limbs.

- Unsteadiness, who always swinging.

- Loss of power

- Diarrhea

- Abnormal Heart pounding, thrill

- A poor heat

- Menstrual Cycle Short

- Weight loss without cause

- Hair loss or hair piece fiber

- Quick blood pulse

- Easy to get excited

- Enlarged thyroid gland.

Where thyroid least, not enough of the hormone the body requires:

- Tired and sleepy during the day

- Dry skin, re

- The voice was hoarse

- Increased weight (weight gain).

- Dry Hair and fall more

- Do not want to eat

- The chills

- On enlargement, particularly puffy eyes, some swelling around the eyes

- Menstrual cycle slow

- Poor memory

- Being constipation

- Thyroid expansion.

Excess or lack of hormones are pathogenic. The disease is difficult or incurable, make patients suffer lifelong disabilities.

However, doctors can intervene in some cases to reduce the disease by means of the medication with radioactive iodide element, or minor surgery to limit the activity of the thyroid gland.

Chapter 3: To keep yourself healthy

You can eat full of nutrients and enough expensive drugs; has quit and spirits, but if you do not exercise the body recommended for athletes, you have the opportunity to just be a somewhat reassuring about his health only. To be healthy, you also need a new generation solid muscle health to preserve, protect new heart and lungs, enhance blood circulation, providing more heat for the body, increase strength containers, made more rigid bones, tendons supple, good digestion, constipation and more no confidence.

Exercise increases the amount of endorphins us- beige, or half a potentially enhanced intellectual resources and human endurance.

Pills can help you cure, less tiring. But want to feel fit to exercise regularly, every day, step by step, starting from today.

Chapter 3 will instruct you how to operate, set goals and exercise program in a specific way in order to protect the health and estimate their progress.

Note: Before entering an exercise program, it is best to consult your health in health care, especially if the previous period day.ban have obesity, high blood pressure, diabetes or heart disease Water . The doctor's advice will help you avoid unnecessary accidents happen during practice, especially on issues related to cardiovascular.

78. Exercise of stress testing

Exercise of stress testing is on purpose to find out how the heart reacts when a person tries to work or exercise. The results of the exercise will help your doctor should advise you how to practice, trying to do the best level that is not harmful to health. If you are going through the stress test exercise, the doctor will ask you to pedal bicycles fixed or take a journey on the go, with the instruments of the heart beat and blood pressure, are mounted in your chest and wrist.

You must necessarily examine exercise it? it depends on your health situation in the past and present. School Sports - American Health, advised people with heart disease or have symptoms of the disease, before joining the training body, should pass the stress test. That's who:

- From 45 years old and had once had symptoms of heart

- Work sedentary

- Have high blood pressure

- Have your blood cholesterol levels (from 240mg / dl or more); 200 - 2400mg / dl: the boundaries of high concentrations; less than 200mg / dl just right: do not worry about heart disease

- Tobacco Addiction

- It results when abnormal EKG

- Have diabetes

- Families with a history of heart disease-related

- There were times when working with chest pain or Campaign

- Has seen tests with cardiovascular disease, lung disease or disorder of metabolism problems.

79. The determination of exercise

Practice or not, depends on the health that depends on the will and your determination. To be able to start training, be dismissed following thoughts out of his mind:

- Training that takes a long time too? Not much. Just 20 to 30 minutes a day. And 5 days a week like that.

- The exercise movements unrelated to what you need. Where no such right. The exercise makes you agile, more lucid mind. Many times, people have devised workarounds work found the answer to every difficult problem in time to take walks.

- The daily exercise really boring leisure!

Boring or not is in him. Today you are cycling, tomorrow, and the day swimming, jogging. Create motphong movement around his workout: with friends, with the husband or wife ..., practicing with many private or group music. Today you bike out gardens, tomorrow to go with his wife and friends to a distance, you have not been to

Make yourself look way this dish, you will never be bored!

80. Set yourself a goal

In anything, if you have a specific goal in mind, you know you have done many things, is some way to go, now you're standing somewhere and so on ...

For bodily exercise their results look like, ask yourself the following questions:

- The results of our practice back home? Pretty, medium or bad? I can train better again? I was at the starting or could escalate even further training?

- I want to improve their health or endurance training, flexibility? One or all three?

- I want to have more to do health? To be better or feel tough, wiser? Or just to prevent disease?

- It should be soon, I reached the goal? is there to achieve?

- With all the daily work to be done, whether we can achieve it?

- There are obstacles to overcome what he? Having overcome it?

- Based on the location where to measure progress? In the weight loss matter? Or based on the number of times fewer colds during the year? On the phenomenon of sleep or less sleep needs first? Or lower cholesterol levels.

- Each time the progress achieved, what I would do to remember or reward? Buy a coat, or going away for your phone?

81. Date with ourselves and kept our word

Every day you have to know how much work to do: to work, to invest, to family ... So how to still be a steady practice? You try to do the following.

- Remember to schedule practice time, as you record any other job you have to.

- Choose exercises that suit the location, the work you're doing at that time the children go to school after lunch before or at the time you have to spend to meet friends and more.

- Choose which do you practice appetite, fun.

- Determined not to give up practicing despite bad sun, cold or busy.

82. The appropriate time

According to surveys of health center southeastern United States in Phoenix, the 75% who workout in the morning after a year, remained sticky practice. While the episode at noon only 50%, and only 25% afternoon. So let's try to get up early, exercise in the morning, before going to work other jobs.

83. Warming up before exercises

Before exercise, always do some warming up, for the muscles get used to the exercise: it is the startup. The launch began gently as the tendons, muscles stretch slowly, not suddenly, to avoid the phenomenon of cramps (muscle cramps), gradually increasing the flow of blood, people-needed heating during exercise in cold weather, winter makes the stretching arms, legs; 5-10 minutes to stretch back stretch

Dynamic stretches:

- Hang arm horizontal, straight up dirt on his head lowered flanks.

- Hang arm -co horizontal hands hand to his chest - to the back of the elbow stretch
- Lower the arm down.

- Put your arms out in front - spinning wrists

- Take up arms before forming the divers feet - before landing and then down. The arm has a horizontal front wing again shrink their shoulders touching.

Back movements. Stand with 2 feet of cage and dirty fingers at each other over his head high. Then raised his head bowed looking at the sky while rotating two hands still knit together, and looking up to the sky, stretching out his hand to the extreme. Hold this for 5 minutes. Slack hands down, to relax, and then redo hand movements stretch 2-4 times.

Leg movements: Title hands on the back of a chair, or on a wall, head straight. A sagging knees slightly while moving it forward and backward. Straight with feet outstretched leg bone to Thoi when feeling tense muscles in the calf. Such Hold for 5 seconds. Lower your foot down and then put your feet up. Redo gestures with the other leg.

When stretching the legs and feet, remember to stretch slowly. When the pain stopped immediately. While stretching, still breathing, not hold your breath.

Want to start fast, warming fast, walk fast a clip, and then run a slow speed. This action makes the heart beat faster and less gradually sweat.

84. Have a break to cool down

5 minute break after the probation period had the opposite effect to when we start, make less body heat and normal again

- Heart gradually returns to normal heartbeat

- The muscle was holiday, reduce tension because where there lactic acid concentration, now that acidity will gradually spread out around them.

- The blood ceased to put down the leg again.

The phenomenon occurs slowly backwards same phenomena startup.

85. Flexible movements

Healthy people need the flexibility of the body, you can practice as follows:

1. Stand with feet firmly 2. Fingers threaded together and put two hands on the head. Keep your hips and leaned fixed very right. Back then tilted into position to the left. 2 remade several times this movement.

2. Sit on the bed or on the floor, legs slightly spread. Keep your back straight, put 2 straight arms to the sky, then bent low in 8-10 seconds. If you feel pain, stop immediately again.

3. Located stretching the legs, back close to the floor slowly bend your knees until thighs onto his right foot pressed into the abdomen and then slowly stretch to on position. Doing this movement with the left leg.

86. The hard moves should be avoided

These movements, if you are not professional sports players, you should avoid, as it may cause back pain.

1. Lie on your back and put your legs over the side, toes touch the floor to the top of the head.

2. Sit astride, arm and tried to bend over.

3. Sitting stretching 2 feet and try to touch your bow is on the toes.

87. Build a table predicting ability to practice

How did your training enough? May set a longer, more severe or moderate strength like that? What is just energy? Volume of about 70-85% of its capacity is moderate. Extreme or excessive collection will be harmful, will make the heart sick. 20-30 minute exercise sessions. 8-4 times per week training (2 days 1 times).

Here is the method for its implementation set for intensity, how time is appropriate to his heart:

1. Before you start, use the right hand left hand pulse (or vice versa). Place the index finger and middle finger up blood vessels in the wrist, gently press down to feel the heartbeat through pulse.

2. Count the number of beats in 10 seconds, (as the clock), then multiply this number 6: This is the normal heart rate for one minute. Example 130

3. After startup movement, amid the collective or immediately after exercise, you manually click back on to the circuit and do the figure recorded her heartbeat for a minute. You choose the highest figure in the last 3 times press circuit. Example: 135

Looking at the table below, find the correct goods listed his age and compare their figures with 135 others in his row to infer such training is slightly longer; is just too much effort or.

- For example: your 40-year-old. After the 20-minute workout, you have the highest heart rate is 135 beats / min. Compared with the safety distances in the table are 128-155. So 135 is smaller than 155 means: you can set more severe.

- If the heart rate after 20 minutes of your set is greater than 155 160: you have to set lighter, or shorten the file. Set 20 minutes before, now only a 15-minute episode.

- If your figures are smaller than the 125 figure at normal beats in Table 128: you have to enhance your walk more to improve his endurance.

After a period of training, the normal heart rate monitors your time will be higher than before: it is a good sign for your health, demonstrating the flexibility of the muscles had improved more.

The table below records the heart rhythm pattern, an American of average health. Better person, there may be other measures than a few ..

About safety heartbeat said measurements at normal heart and after training, in the range that has proved to collective effort, has used about 70-85% of their capacity.

88. What benefit Walk?

Walking is a method of maintaining health that anyone can perform. Walking has the following benefits:

- How the heart and blood circulation faster circuits

- Increases the body's heat

- Increases strength and muscle endurance

- Increases the body's stamina

- Easy digestion and are

- The blood pressure

- Feeling Healthy

When walking up:

- Go slow at first 2-3 minutes, as the startup time

- Before and after, should sit 2-3 minutes of legroom

- Shoes should match the leg

- When you step heel down first and then set bend the toes walk.

- When going to keep a straight posture, head slightly raised, shoulders incense swinging arm in the direction of the hit.

- Inhale deeply and exhale all

- Before the stop, slow down for 3-5 minutes.

89. Cycling is useful for health

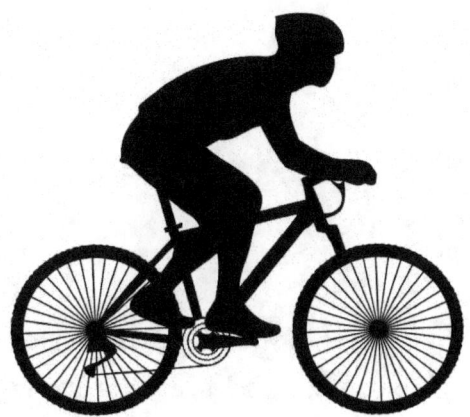

Cycling is good for both body and spirit because you can go to places with fresh air, which increases the blood flow and you will feel better. No need to pedal as fast as the racers. Here are the measures to prevent leg cramps and sore muscles:

- Handles and seat cushion to suit your height. It is best to adjust the saddle How to be at full stretch when cycling.

- When the bike arrived, should have at minute break to stretch the arms, legs, back. Before cycling and so on.

90. Under-water exercises

In the water, you see people as light as a leaf. If you swim, you will feel his weight dropped to 90%. You can gently move the bones, muscles, elbows and feet, knees and back vertebra comfortable movement. Many athletes on the difficult but saw arms, legs ... easy movement while under water, in the pool or ... in the bathtub. Advocacy underwater fits:

- People over 50 years old

- The joint pain

- Painful calf or back pain.

91. Can you swim cross the Atlantic?

In the water, you see as light as a leaf. If you swim, you feel his weight dropped to 90%. You can gently move the bones, muscles, elbows and feet, knees and back vertebra comfortable movement. Athletes on the difficult but many saw arms, legs ... easy movement while under water, in the pool or in the bathtub.... Advocacy underwater fits:

- People over 50 years old

- The joint pain

- Painful calf or back pain.

92. What is Aerobic?

Keep the balance of your arms, legs, body movement and the beat: it is the practice of aerobic. In such context, running, or cycling can also considered aerobic, such as aerobics. When aerobic exercise, our heart and lungs have to work from 60 to 85% of their capacity.

From about 1980, the exercise becomes rhythmic movement but many people jump and bend over, have caused many problems and affect bone and tendons.

Today, it has been reorganizing too strong movements while volumes have avoided the accident. To this must be remembered when the file:

- Only put one foot off the ground. One foot always touching the floor.

- Limit 2 foot jump all at once

- Restrict movements startle

Gentle aerobic type, require the collective

- Do not jump 2 feet at a time

- The movements in all major sports and large muscles (such as biceps, thighs), sedentary small muscles (such as the feet, wrists ...)

- Advocating arms than the other.

93. What is a good Aerobic class?

What Aerobics class is good and right for you? Name each of the following questions and answers:

1. Aerobic teacher certification is equal or coach

School, sports center or institute yet or not?

2. Floor internship sure? Do not practice on mats or carpets thin: very susceptible to slip.

3. Gym with air conditioners?

4- The room caters for people from the collision set it?

5. Startup time and rest every episode has a habit yet?

6. Each time set to 20 minutes it?

7. You may be instructed to count your pulse before, during, and after exercise does not

8. You get to spend a comfortable place for himself during practice it?

9- The coach has put the new routines and new tunes into not exercising.

10. After training, you can feel comfortable and healthy people to it? Or feel that something is not right?

Depending on the number of times you answered "yes", you evaluate aerobic classes are suitable for you or not.

94. Select the appropriate practice to body

Health state of everyone is different. Bone structure, muscles, tendons, too. So, each person has an appropriate number of private practice. Example:

Type 1, including those who seem to look:

- Chubby, round, smooth shape

Do not exercise much jump all requirements.

Up: walking, cycling, swimming and gentle exercises little twisted, twisted person

Type 2, including those who:

- Bones to, many muscles

- Broad shoulders, chest

- On seems to "fill power"

Up: walking, running short distances (5 km return)

Do not: Running the marathon, a training session with the game, the exercise requires balance, health and ingenuity (tennis or sailing)

Type 3, including but people:

- High, Long Neck

- Shoulders, narrow hips, small breasts

- Long limbs

- Wrist, small footprint

- The small, slightly fat

- In practice, hard muscles

Not suitable subjects: swimming and running quickly.

Suitable for subjects: basketball, tennis, running tough.

95. Train in accordance with human

The practice is not only based on the figure, but also depends on the individual streak. Some people prefer collective crowded places, outdoor, people prefer to have it alone in the house ... So, if you can choose the practice suit individual interests, the collective is more enjoyable.

There are people every weekend to keep boiling should be named

"The soldier weekend." If you have the same blood, should participate in practice require endurance (distance cycling, football, basketball, marathon...), and noted with care to avoid accidents because of their "enthusiasm "too.

Who are "fanatical". With these, the episode has just as good, but much better practice. They are suited to avail sport, requires effort. Long warm memories when they fail. Should advise them: sport is entertainment, not so bitter!

Type "Butterflies": Interest join the many people practice and changing practice. Coach's advice: when practicing, so trust in yourself is key, so do not rely on other people too much.

Type "ephemeral": very enthusiastic at first but easy to give up

Tips: The results obtained only exercise 10 to 12 weeks. Should strive for 2- 3 weeks did not affect how much health.

Type "Theory": Like collecting all sorts of books and materials about the sport. Join what does it cost half the money to buy all kinds of instruments on that subject. Or presentation of your friends all the benefits and advantages of their collective goal.

Tip: try to practice what you are 50% for reading.

96. Choose a progress for yourself

If you do not choose your progress carefully, you will easily give up halfway. In addition to the main practice should have some extra practice instead. For example, you used to play tennis with a friend. Have expected the other day absent friend, what would you do? I'll be walking, cycling, swimming or basketball throw?

Excluding advance so easily give up practicing in vain stiffened sitting in a coffee shop.

97. Statistical Tabulation his progress

After a probationary period, whether the health had got better or not? How many kilograms has been contracted? Hips, chest than before is how much? Do I sleep better before? There is no better feeling?

All these things can be neatly defined method: measuring heart rate after resting.

Some as small resting heart rate, proved better health. Therefore, if your practice is the result of the measured heart rate at rest, will be smaller than before.

Measuring as before:

1 - Press your circuit at dawn, as he got up, got out of bed yet.

2. Count your pulse for 10 seconds and then multiply by 6, you get the pulse for 1 minute.

3. The next morning the press again. Plus the number of pulse twice, then split, taking the average pulse.

Three months at a time. If files are, you will see the circuit is reduced, said your health has increased.

98. Over-working

Are you over-working or not? After the training session, if you find yourself talking to other people to breathe more difficult because, embarrassed if someone invited to go dancing or walking distances drooping, then maybe you overdo it. You must file away or stop the exercise at a time to recharge.

99. 3 abdominal exercises to burn fat

If you lose belly fat of 2-4kg, there will be less concern on excess cholesterol, high blood pressure and blood sugar balance. Here are some jerks the abdominal muscles, you select the action that you feel suits you.

Problem 1. Fold the head and neck - Lie on your back, leg curl, both hands to the lower head. Keeping your back against the floor, try to lift your head and shoulders about 30 degrees.

Note: Keep your head, neck and spine in a straight line. As the group slowly, inhale and count to 5 and then slowly lay down. Redo this movement 10-15 times you will see the effect on the muscles in the abdomen.

Lesson 2. folding of the hands, sitting teach - In back, knees bent, arms crossed over his chest, his right hand holding his left shoulder, left hand holding his right shoulder all.

Bend to sit up, then lay down again from 10-15 times.

Problem 3. Hands back of the neck, sitting got up - hands to the lower spine, fingers laced together. Lie on your back with knees bent, feet slightly away from each other. Sat curled up, touched his right hand to his left knee. Lie down, got up, hit the left elbow to right knee. (While this action does not last note 2 first hand forward) Do movements 10-15 times.

100. The exercise apparatus

Instruments: go, running in place, cycling, turned ... to pull parts, belts, bikes, etc ... installed hook at home, is the collective instruments are many people dream. However, before you buy, you must understand the effects of each type of instrument for instruments including matching your needs. For example, stationary bike tools work to lower body and heart, but has no effect to the hands and not do a tummy.

Therefore, before you buy to think to their collective purpose in order not to "quickly bored" with instruments and should:

- Find out which vendors and stores selling instruments sound or 'no.

- Ask friends who have used this device for features and tools to buy where.

- Considering the price is right for my pocketbook

- Try before paying instruments

- Seeing how instruments assemble, move the star, where the placement, consistent with their circumstances do not ... Ask a tool storage like.

- Requires tools must be warranted.

- Think again considered himself set with tools like this not to escape quickly bored.

101. Choose the right shoes

Carpenters need compatriots, miners need shovels, do also need specialized tools such as mechanic. Good tools are also easily add jobs. His Shoes exercise or play sports, too. It can make you comfortable or uncomfortable, get you safe or for which the accident occurred, it can contribute to the achievement of your company or not.

Therefore, before you begin, you must select the proper shoes for your feet and ask yourself:

- Shoes are suitable for my practice? As per the practice, such as travel, bike, baseball, tennis, aerobics ... requires shoes with different characteristics.

- I have to stand up at the toe of the shoe stand and when to sit it? (To stand up).

- Width of shoes available in horizontal vacuum? (Grab the pencil lines under 2 feet when standing on the edge and then measured as above 2 next shoe with a colored pencil. If greater dimensional two-dimensional edge 2 foot shoe edge, then the shoes, the foot will be limited).

- The seams in his shoes with heels made uncomfortable? (do not be like that). When removing the shoe, the upper can be squashed down to zero? (not)

- When going all been tight shoes with it? (not)

- When traveling, dancing, shoes match the vacuum? (You try and jump before you buy)

Good pair of shoes is the shoes make you comfortable right from carrying it on foot, for the first time.

102. What to do with the weather?

You lucky to be anywhere there are many seasons, because you can change the practice to suit the weather. Thus, the practice will be richer, support boring. However, you can comment as to keep some for his experience on the selection of the practice: the practice has enjoyed over the summer, but became illegal or dangerous in winter.

When winter sets in, should:

- Wear pants, long shirt to cover wind and moisture resistant, cold.

- Wear a hat. No hat or scarf to cover his head, you can lose up to 40% of the first heat during training

- Wear lightweight jacket warmer 3-5 2 thick coat. Do not wear clothing with quality polypropylene (raincoat fabric), because of the type of clothing like moisturizing and will eventually cause you to be cold. In the beginning, to walk or run into the wind to time to go running with the wind. At this point, you have sweating, running against the wind prone to colds.

- It runs in the road because the floor will house the wind cover for you.

- Do not smoke and drink coffee or alcohol, because the things that make you cold again.

In the summer, should:

- Wear lightweight, easy to waterproof. Do not wear long pants, long coat and waterproof fabrics do hard sweat evaporation.

- Wearing glasses to avoid sun glare

- Start training slowly

- Before training as well as during practice, should drink plenty of fluids, even if you are not thirsty.

- It should be set at the coolest time of day - early morning - or afternoon - when the sun absence.

103. Practice, should eat better

During exercise, you need to have diet and drink well.

The substances of hydrogen - carbon cake, flour, potatoes ... and fruit give you energy needed for exercise. But do not rush to eat just before practice. You have to eat earlier from one to two hours. But foods like bread milk, bread, banana and a glass of orange juice will contribute positively to the achievement of his your workout.

104. Time to eat?

Exercise then eat or eat then exercise? Why do you need to pay attention to this issue?

- Do not eat right before practice because during practice, most of the blood was put to the muscles. Your digestive parts unnoticed to be a lack of energy to operate. Therefore, should aim for 2-3 hours after a meal and 1-2 hours after a light meal.

- Keep all breakfast diet. Before you set the morning, before breakfast, you can eat a cake form, drink a glass of juice before the training field 15-20 minutes.

- If you train in the afternoon, to eat lunch and dinner a bit late.

105. What to do when aching joints?

Aching joints in arms, legs, joint pain, muscle aches ... is often seen in exercise or sports. When the pain you still trying to practice or play continued, the pain can last for weeks or months.

When you see the pain, should:

- Stay and pay attention not to the sore must operate within 24-48 hours.

- Apply cold water or ice from 5-20 minutes per hour, within 2-3 days, until the feeling of pain and pain do not see hot to touch.

- Secure with elastic bandage pain well, for 30 minutes. Remove the tape and then tied back on in 15 minutes. Doing so repeatedly.

- When sleeping or lying, higher pain Statistics.

If necessary, take aspirin for pain, with plenty of water or milk to avoid the negative effects of aspinn to stomach.

Should consult a doctor if:

- Pain or stride, heavy hands.

- There is numbness identical phenomenon.

- Skin packaging bruised place.

- The bones are misaligned bridles together.

- Do not move because of pain.

106. Stop exercising when you are sick?

There are many charismatic practices of ours that make the flu, sore throat, colds, fever ... we did not want to leave. Doing something that is not helpful to us all.

Ie had a fever when our body is not stabilized. If we re-set the body tired easy to do more, give us health to burnout, creating favorable conditions for the disease to appear. If you have a cold, stop the exercise again. For the exercise to enhance the circulation of blood this time just bad. The bacteria or virus is carried by the blood to every point in the body faster than normal. In contrast, the stop practicing for two or three days will help you to restore health to the back training, will find more affinity.

Chapter 4: Food and Health

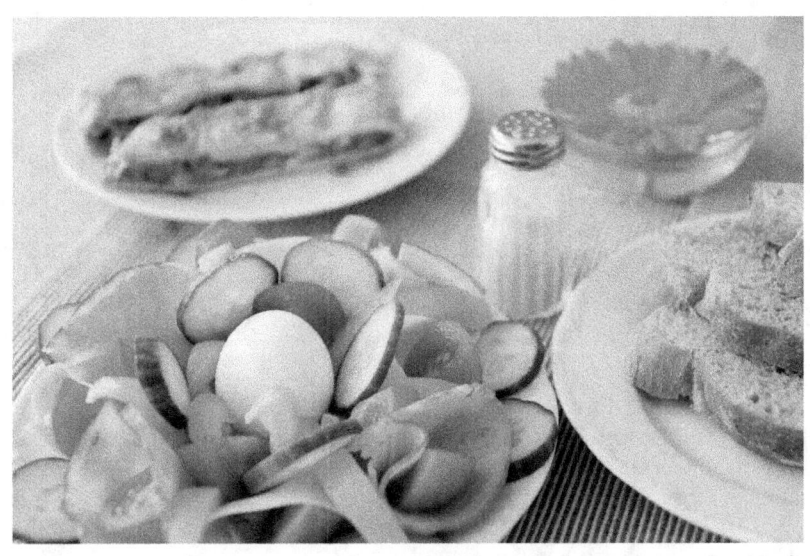

Many researchers have said about food: beta-carotene is found in RNO boy, pumpkin, orange, yellow skin and some vegetables could help the body to slow Gaya cancer. They also are a good source of vitamin A is necessary for the body. But foods with fiber is not only good for digestion but also contribute to removing bile acids in the bile in the food passes through the intestine, avoiding the formation of gallstones evidence and colon cancer. Many tests have proven that people who eat a lot of tuna, salmon and many other fish that are high in omega fatty acids types - 3, has reduced the amount of triglycoride and blood cholesterol.

The above is the news that the press always refers to raise the importance of choosing foods for meals.

This book chapters you want with statistics foods rich in vitamins, and nutrients to the choice, put on the meal to increase your health and your family.

107. Differences between fruits and juices

Have you ever drank a bottle of orange juice, just ask the question: on what nutritional differences between drinking bottle of orange juice and eat an orange?

Bottle of orange juice can contain more vitamin C, soda - do digestible substance gas and a number of substances present in wine

Fresh oranges also contain

- Many more orange substance

- Creates less energy

- There are many fiber.

The research in the laboratory said fiber in the fruit only, but not in the juice or juice. Fiber contribute regulate substances -cacbon hydrogen and metabolism in the body. Fruit sugars are absorbed by the body more slowly than sugar in the juice. The phenomenon of sugars in the body moved slowly into the blood is a good thing because such things, the amount of insulin in the body and is released slowly to keep blood sugar levels stable and people feel more comfortable.

Remember, most of the juice of the fruit contains very little that only water, sweeteners, flavorings and colorants alone! So: better eating oranges orange juice drink!

108. Select and preserve vegetables and fruit?

Fruits and vegetables are the "warehouse" foods full of vitamins. Should buy, select and hold fruits like?

- Choose the left to see firm and glossy. Choose vegetables, too.

- For the lemon and pineapple, choose fruit firm and heavy (relative to volume).

- Do not buy, but the fruit was dark and mushy.

- Do not buy too much redundancy or capacity to store vegetables in the refrigerator compartment. Do not buy a lot of extra lemon and orange because you can buy an extra food but can not eat bananas to add a lemon.

- Not long soak in water.

- Sprinkling mild dry after washing.

- These fruits are rich in vitamin C such as oranges, lemons easily damaged when exposed to air. Therefore, never eat freshly cut.

109. Indicators of vitamin minor

Signage below includes some typical food linked to a number of vitamins. Also remember that the food does not have the ability to provide all of the vitamins that our body needs, especially in special cases, such as pregnant women, menstruating, seconded patients dieting, people with allergies etc .. in such conditions, it is necessary to add supplements and vitamins is formulated.

110. A number of metallic elements in food

The metallic elements such as calcium (Ca), iron (Fe), zinc (Zn) are essential for the body as well as vitamins. The table below tells us that the effects of the elements that the body and the food that contains the metallic element useful.

As with vitamins, the special conditions of the bodies of pregnant women, menstruation, illness, to dieting, food allergies ... need to take that to provide enough power metal necessary for the body.

111. Why must wash?

You often remind young children: "Wash your hands before eating." Particularly adults, not just wash your hands often more careful, wash all the food you eat. This excess is not? Not. Because farmers often use fertilizers, pesticides or drugs etc ... in general are toxic chemicals co'the human hooves, to fertilize and protect the crop. It is clear that such chemicals remain on each leaf vegetables, fruit peel that we bought, and none of us want to eat all kinds of chemicals that. you need to remember:

- We should buy the food produced in the country, since the tests showed vegetables, fruit imported from abroad are often more contaminated vegetables

- Be careful when you eat peaches, celery, lettuce, strawberries. These fruits and vegetables are often contaminated more than other types of chemicals, such as corn, cauliflower, banana, cucumber.

- Wash fruits and vegetables with diluted soapy water. Combed and dry.

112. What is beneficial for bones to eat?

Many adults think the age has stopped the development of bone tissue, ie deactivated. Think so are wrong! Old bone cells always be replaced with newborn cells eat enough material to provide for the regeneration of new bone cells, which are the issues to consider when eating throughout the our life. Calcium is a metallic element most abundant in the human body, but the body was not homemade. Therefore we have to eat the food there for- to give poker body. Milk and dairy products also contain Viatmin D and some other substance that helps the body to absorb easily Can - xi.

Green leafy vegetables, legumes, fruits, cereals, sardines, salmon ... eat the bones, are rich foods Can - cement, mainly elemental bone growth and tough measures. Children aged 1 to 10 years of age take 800 mg shifts / day; 11-18 years old:

1200 mg / day; 18 and older: 800 mg / day. Pregnant women and breastfeeding:

1,200 - 1.600mg / day.

113. Who cannot use milk?

Millions of people on earth are easy to drink milk. Yet there are people "hydrophobic milk". Why? Because their digestive system is not sold lactose in milk and milk products. Just as they were eaten:

- Flatulence in the lower abdomen (the large intestine)

- Stomachache

- Face puffy and allergies

- Diarrhea

- Nausea, vomiting.

The intestinal diseases occur when drinking milk or eating a cake milk, a piece of cheese - ... Only after a few minutes and lasts for hours due to lack of parts digestive enzymes to digest lactose in milk. Because milk is a very good nutrition, rich elemental calcium - so if they are going without milk and dairy products used, the body will lose a source of vital energy.

Therefore, the "hydrophobic milk" should:

- Fasting the cakes yet his body reaction or an eating small amounts. Avoid milk and dairy products in solid, concentrated.

- Mix the milk with lactase enzymes are usually named in pharmacy sold in powder or also called Lactaid members. Lactase mixing into milk 24 hours before drinking. Lactase tablets can be used as digestive aids drugs.

- Looking to buy milk and products such as ice cream, cheese - specially prepared with Lactase is often sold in the super-rich foods Can thi.a - cement, mainly elemental bone growth and tough measures. Children aged 1 to 10 years of age take 800 mg shifts / day; 11-18 years old:

1200 mg / day; 18 and older: 800 mg / day. Pregnant women and breastfeeding:

1,200 - 1.600mg / day.

114. Why eat fiber?

It may seem strange to say a sentence as follows: "Fiber is not food but also the food". Why has not, has there? Not the food because the digestive apparatus of us do not spend is fiber intake and go out, eat fiber we avoid constipation disease lowers blood cholesterol levels and prevent cancer. Thus the fiber present in the seeds and crops - obviously very useful for human health.

Commission Food and Drug Administration (FDA) of the United States suggest each of us eat from 25-30g of fiber per day in fruits, vegetables, beans and grains series. It distinguishes two types of fiber: soluble and insoluble. The cakes are high in fiber, which acts as lowering cholesterol, made of:

- Barley mixed with bran.

- Dry beans and legumes.

- Oat bran.

What kind of rear wheels that contain insoluble fibers, is effective against constipation and cancer orders, made of:

- Flour corn.

- Some legume.

- Wheat bran.

- Left nodes.

Many fruits, vegetables, legumes and nuts contain both soluble and insoluble fiber in the country. Changing food is making delicious meals because exotic, and provide food for the body to have both types of fiber.

115. How to eat meat?

Many people hesitate to eat meat because meat - especially fatty meat - is the "culprit" causing many diseases. Therefore they abstain from all meat foods such as steak, hamburger ... and switch to chicken, duck and fish. According to the agency's report, the current US agriculture, due attention in livestock breeding and meat classified as selling, people have had these types of pork and beef without fat or very fat compared with all kinds of pork and beef 25 years ago.

It's a good news for red meat protein source is important, rich in iron, zinc, man - liver and vitamin B category as thia min, riboflavin, niacin and.

You can safely eat without fear of excessive weight gain, increased cholesterol and heart disease. But also need to pay attention to the following points?

- When shopping, choose a good meat

- Eat lunch just right, do not eat more contact - Crawler

- Notice the careful selection of sausages for many types of advertising are not effective as a fat, leaving not enough nutrients because it contains a lot of water and mix pointless.

- Comb additional brown fat meat before

- Better Barbecue or fried fries

- Every time you eat meat do not eat more than 3-5 ounces (oz = 18.25 g)

- Each week should only eat 5 times.

116. Use marinated meats like?

Salted meats, smoked meats, sausages etc ... have been salted, or potassium - nitrate, sulfur smoked or cooked by firewood to prevent bacteria reside and development. Many scientists believe that nitrite and nitrate salts, keep the meat is not broken but can be switched to nitrosamines is a substance capable of causing cancer. But really lucky because of Vitamin C could prevent metabolic above. Therefore, the ham processors have more vitamin C attention to the composition of substances used to preserve raw meat.

When we use the marinated meats or smoked meats, note:

- Salted or roasted meat can still be broken because stale, rotten at normal temperature. Therefore, the right to the refrigerator.

- If possible, before using it for a few minutes in the oven meat ultrasound because the furnace is capable of killing bacteria.

- When cooking meat, the more fat to be soaked when dripping fat, will reduce the rate of soluble and nitrosamines (if any).

Also note that these meats contain a lot of fat and salt. Therefore, should limit fat and soot. Therefore, it should be limited.

117. Should not eat barbecue?

In summer, many Americans like to participate in outdoor meals with pork, lamb, beef ... grilled over charcoal, gas or electric stove stove. These delicious dishes that fit both custom properties, but unfortunately some scientists considered very dangerous for health.

National Academy of Sciences said, so there may be a link between the grilled food and cancer. Some studies suggest that the fat and protein - in corruption and protein foods contain more fat as ham - burger, for example, when being grilled at high temperatures easily converted into mutagens, are chemicals capable of destroying jealous system of cells in the body and lead to cancer. While these opinions have not been formally recognized right or wrong, we should also precaution, do not always eat barbecue. When food or barbecue, should follow some instructions:

- Before grilling meat (pork, beef, chicken, duck or fish), should remove the fat out. Do not immerse the meat in fat, butter or oil before baking.

Poultry prepared ready to spray sprays water into the meat when the meat of ignition

- When baking, meat ho above heat source, over the fire

- If the fire is too strong to be quenching furnace or lower heat away.

If not, then transfer the meat to the side of the fire.

- Bake for cooked meat but avoid very charred meat because dogs charred to a cinder, but that might be the cause.

- Avoid fire grilled fish and vegetables wrapped outside. So pack the meat in aluminum foil.

- Before baking, the meat in the oven up to ultrasound to reduce the amount of fat and shorten the baking time.

118. Always eat fish

Research on diet Eskimos - a people northernmost ó! A bridge, it was found that despite eating a lot of fat, very few people with heart disease Eskimos. The reason health so, because in addition to fat, this nation also eat a lot of fish. These fish live in cold waters such as mackerel, salmon contains lots of omega fatty acids

- 3 in the flesh, is very beneficial for health

- To reduce cholesterol and blood fats as triglyxerid. Avoid blood clots in the vessels

- Making the breast tumor (if any), retardation

- To support the headaches

- To support joint pain.

Omega-3 is found in fish and other seafood, is easily absorbed by the body through the gastrointestinal tract. Therefore, each week we should eat fish or other seafood from 2-4 times as:

- The male

- Arctic Cod

- Pink salmon

- Herring

- Trout live in the lake

- Isaac-đin fish (sardin)

- Pilchard

119. Water is essential for cell

Two-thirds of our body is liquid water which is the main component. Therefore, water plays a very important role to give the body the necessary metal elements such as Can - xi and Ma - magnetite.

- Helps the body absorb and digest essential food easily.

- Putting the nutrients in the blood to go everywhere in the body.

- Making oily membrane tissues and joints.

- Helps the body of waste residue.

- Controls body heat escape sweat band phenomenon.

Many people do not pay enough attention to the need to drink water. Adults should drink 6-8 glasses of water every day.

We can coordinate the food and water intake in foods:

- Lettuce (containing 95% water).

- Cantaloupe (containing 91% water)

- Radish contains (88% water)

120. What is the benefit of eating soup?

Soup is good for healthy. When sick sinus or cold, cold, very good chicken soup. Why can lose weight eating soup?

Because each muonng drank until all the soup usually takes more time to eat an equivalent amount of nutrients in the form of solid or solid food for so long, the brain feels lease agreements and severance hunger or food cravings anymore . While eating a hamburger pieces done, the brain is still developing may ask: "Only that's all?"

Here are some more nutritious soup: shrimp soup with more calcium -, vitamin D and protein than milk soup.

Soup with vegetables, beans and rice are substances that make the fiber more easily digested.

- When cooking vegetable soup for less water when cooking meat soup. (For vegetables that release of water).

- Be sure to spice up the soup with herbs such as parsley, onion powder, garlic powder instead of salt.

121. Eat less salt!

When there was no refrigerator, then salted food is the most convenient method, it is often used to store food for long. Things that are not good for health because some people eat salt can lead to high blood pressure, heart attack, stroke and edema. Salt we eat out of habit rather than by innate need. So if now we do not eat more salt or salt substitute with a substance other spices in meals is also no harm to health at all.

Here are some ideas:

- Let the salt shaker away from the kitchen and the dining table so you can forget about it.

- When adding spices to food, cooking, use less salt and salty condiments.

- When buying food even should buy a light.

- Avoid buying foods such as pickled cucumber, olives, vinegar and other improvements

- Limit your intake of salted fish, salted meat.

- What to buy fresh meat for cooking instead of buying food

- When eating out, should call clearly less salt foods.

We fasted much salt because salt contains up to 40% Natrium element is the element does not affect health benefits, and is related to some diseases for the elderly.

122. Select what type of meat?

If the market has only certain types of fresh meat, there's no problem for us to comment. But according to the advertisement, there are many kinds of meat marinated mu- attacks, cinnamon marinated fish, meat tri sodium levels low, moderate sugar content etc. These endorsements in fact, only generic without clear, about a problem at all. When buying meat, we need to ask to know:

- The amount of meat in the package is much, small or big pieces?

- Number of packaging.

- Value of how many calories in calories?

- Contains how much protein, fat, hydrogen carbide, specific provisions of grams.

- Contains many Natrium, equivalent in milligrams

- Contains many vitamins and metallic elements what?

Some good fliers said clearly rules out milligrams cholesterol. Here are some of our conventions need to understand the content. If there is any doubt on the ad: meats

- The amount of low calorie means: 40 cal/ 100g.

- Number of calories restriction: only 1/3 calories than other meats.

- Meat particularly sodium and sugars limited.

- Low sodium content: contains about 35 mg of sodium or less.

- Less fat: less fat contains 10-25% less than other types.

123. Strategy for reducing fat and cholesterol in the food

The coronary artery disease is the disease of the heart making many Americans die prematurely. The cause of the disease is the deposition of fat and cholesterol in the arteries, especially in the heart vessels. Therefore, we need to know a number of measures to reduce the amount of fat and cholesterol in the diet.

- When boiling or drinking milk, fat cottage away.

- Decrease meat and eggs, only eat 5-7 times a week.

- Eat eggs according to the formula: 1 time 2 times give away the whites and yolks.

- Trim the fat off meat before cooking. If you eat chicken, duck, then remove the skin.

- Do not eat fried meat, especially smoked meats, bacon, chicken, fish duck.

- Take them away fat floating on the soup before serving

- Cooked eggs, fish with water than doing the dishes with butter.

- Use a frying pan specially without lube.

- When needed, use fat instead of fat herb oil and margarine instead of butter.

- Limiting the required mix of oil, grease and replace it with the vinegar or lemon juice mixed with food.

- The use of olive oil as fat because this oil can combat heart disease properties. Canola oil, too.

- Limit or do not eat meat, fish fried butter.

124. The good edible oils

Some oils have the potential to reduce cholesterol in the body. However, you should only use from 5-8 teaspoons of them per day for each subject: cooking, frying, mixed vegetables etc.

- Oil wealth

- Corn beans

- Olive oil

- Peanuts

- Sesame oil

- Soybean Oil.

125. Eating method to avoid cancer

Several studies have said the food and drink was the cause of 60% of cases of cancer in women and 30-40% cases in men.

But it is difficult to say, we should eat or not to eat anything. The scientists recommend that we should follow only a few things are as follows:

- Eat less fat. Therefore, to limit the types of beef, pork, butter, cream, cheese - coconut oil and oils hydrogien.

- Eat more vegetables, fruits, bread made from whole grains. Foods rich in beta - carotene, carrots, potatoes, vegetables, dark green color or gold seems likely to help the body fight cancer. Vitamin C-rich fruits such as lemon, melon, tomatoes are good for the stomach and the esophagus, allowing these parts to avoid the disease.

Fiber foods can also help cancer restrictions such as seeds of cereals, vegetable foods: legumes, cabbage, asparagus ... It is assumed that in the composition of foods it also has some vitamins and some anti-cancer agents that one unidentified

- Avoid eating meat kebabs marinated and smoked meats such as meat containing nitrite and nitrate can cause cancer stem stomach and esophagus.

- Drink little or no alcohol is best. Along with tobacco, which both enjoy oral cancer, throat and esophagus. They are the causes of breast cancer disease and liver cancer.

For the Americans, drinking in moderation is 1- 2 doses per day. Every time you drink, do not exceed 12 ounces of beer, 5 ounces of wine, and 0.5 ounces of spirits such as Vodka, whiskey (1 ounce = 28.35 g).

126. Eat breakfast before work

Can we assure, if we start a machine to run without refueling the vehicle? Yet many people omit the breakfast before going to work. Some scientists have noticed the reduction of manual labor led the corner who does not mind working to achieve high efficiency in those days they did not eat breakfast in the morning.

If you do not feel like eating at the new up, try to follow the following measures:

- Think before her breakfast dishes from the night before. Thus, you should take time to think once stark wake up and brush your teeth.

- Pack the breakfast things in a small package the night before, so the next day to eat on the way to school or to the office: a few small loaves, some cheese and fruits.

- Change the dishes away. Do not always eat the same day. This will cause her to anorexia.

- If you feel you lose your appetite, try eating less one can eat fruit or vitamin C in the early morning, such as strawberry, grape, orange, etc.

These protein-rich foods will make you sober. Therefore, a better glass of milk glass of juice. A piece of bread than a piece of apple. Avoid ham, sausage, eggs are rich in fatty substances and cholesterol. Nor should eat fresh bread, pies, cakes and fat-rich sugars.

127. Establish a healthy eating habit

Building for your child a healthy eating habit is essential. Here are the main points:

- Morning for children up hot bread breakfast cereal made better all sweets, although she likes more.

- Give children foods with low levels of fat, sugar and salt. Fresh fruit, baked goods from food grain, milk, juice, yogurt are all good nutrients.

- Limit the "snacks" buy at the store. The buy-eat dishes, often fat and not enough nutrients.

- Do not take food as reward measures, phat.Neu fined, they will be missing nutrients to the body and if rewarded, they will not have the discipline to eat and sometimes eat too full.

- Want your child has an eating routine, the supply to such parents to set an example.

- If the children have lunch at school, they can prepare for the children bring from home:

- Burgers meat - sandwiches with chicken, avocado, cheese, tuna. On vegetables and fruits can make sure they carry grape, apple, tomato - chopped carrot, celery stalk. Jam jar food is also easy to carry.

- Also note the children that juice bottle is much less water flavored with sugar and food coloring.

- The pastries in the shop more often and less nutritious sugar.

- The salt cake is soaked with oil, salt and coloring, not enough nutrients in foods brought from home.

As for the age of 13-14 onwards, need special attention because of large skeleton fast requires lots of Can - xi. The granddaughter also need iron, because every time menstrual blood loss grandchildren.

- Fried chicken leg is provided iron dish.

- Low fat milk, yogurt, cheese, etc.

- Cantaloupe, Cucumber and eat fruit instead of vegetables are very good for this age group.

128. What should be ordered in a quick meal?

Every day, 50 million Americans often go to the "fast food" restaurant. Mostly, they call three main dishes: hamburgers, fries and milk shakes. Many people do not know that now in the places that people sell vegetables coleslaw, fries, soups and snacks in the store, so:

- Avoid fried meats. Better to eat barbecue.

- If you have to order omelets, may propose replaced by pasta with sauce onion, mushroom pepper.

- Instead of dipping sauce a la carte, so called salad and fresh fruit.

- Eat barbecue should eat lettuce.

- Can be replaced by mu- attacks.

- Low fat milk, fresh fruit juice or water, rather than regular milk and soft drinks

- If the milk into the coffee - coffee, also use low-fat milk.

129. What is the food processed through radiation?

In the supermarket stores, packages of food like vegetables, fruit have outside envelope with a stamp of "radiation". What does that mean?

The method compares the radiation, a type of radiation can kill the bacteria that spoil food - is a method of branches Food and Drug Is approval for widespread application in the food industry and in society. Food is irradiated with radiation is not lost or saved odor residue, no chemicals that need to retain long not broken. Radiation can kill germs and bacteria without food nutrients lost. The study also demonstrated this kind of radiation is not related to cancer and harmless to human health.

Chapter 5: Tips to lose weight - control your weight

According to the investigation by health care organizations and people of the United States, 37% of Americans get their desired weight loss. Among those who want to slim down so, with 27% male and 47% female.

It is calculated that there are 60 million Americans are overweight. Anthem Why so?

Because newspapers and television ads full of all sorts of food. Fast food, snacks, ubiquitous. There are many types of bread with nutty flavor, but too much food because appetite is one thing everyone can do easily.

People who are overweight may be prey Crab several diseases such as hypertension, diabetes, heart disease and so on ... So how to curb eating is an important issue.

In this chapter you will be introduced to self-control measures in the food problem, know how choose delicious foods that fit no more than 100 calories, while eating at a hotel, we do not much fat carte , should set yourself how diet during breaks etc.

In short, how to lose weight, the body and the weight just right, as you wish.

130. The ideal weight

We often compare our weight with the weight of others to see who has the balance just right. In fact, the comparison that makes no sense if the two high, low different. S staining ideal weight should fit both height again. Through the following sample table, you will need to figure out your workout to keep some weight, to gain weight or lose weight.

131. Try seeing whether your waist excesses fat

Many people wonder if they have heavy excess, and depending on the type of fat balance? For this, you need to clearly account for how much fat percentage of body weight. Here is how to proceed to determine the matter.

Making testing by Pinch (Profiles): Pinch (structure) into the skin in three points:

- On the upper arm

- Between the thighs

- Besides the belly.

Use of multi-thickness measurement. Mentioned thickness skin pinched up from 1 inch measured or less (inch - 25 mm) lower your fat or at the average.

If greater thickness of the skin, then every 1/4 inch (0.5 mm) is 4,5kg excess fat.

Trying as above, helps you keep track of the weight or spend your dream while you are eating under the special regime or practice, for the purpose of going the extra fat and weight monitoring. If your body does not have that excess fat weight, reduction was demonstrated in muscles working. If so should decrease and increase the training set up.

132. Set for yourself the amount of weight to lose

If you want to drop 7kg, 10kg or 15kg in a year in which new sales decreased 3 - 4kg, do not be discouraged. The problem is not the practice to no avail but because you have set high targets too. Now, you should set up again with a smaller, more easily achieved and in a shorter time limit.

For example, think that I will try to set for the following three weeks, fell by 2kg. After falling by 2kg, you set yourself back at practice to be 2kg more falling, which continued like that until the goal is reached 10kg, 15kg.

Small-turn and go to where they also specify that jobs seem to perform better.

133. How many calories do you need to provide per day?

Calculate the amount of heat to the body of calories you need each day, equivalent to the weight of friends. Therefore, you need to know each day I have to eat as much to provide sufficient number of calories your body needs. To do so, you must follow these steps:

1. Consider the sample table of ideal weight to choose the weight just right for you.

2. For example, you find yourself suited to the weight of 130 pounds. (Pounds = 0,455kg).

3. If you are the activities (biking, walking, swimming several times a week ...) you multiply the number 130 for 9 (130 x 9 = 1.170). So you need 1,170 calories per day.

If you are decommissioned more (join aerobics tennis, reaquet ...) Human 130 x 10, so that you need, 1,300 calories / day.

If you are sedentary (sitting sewing, reading, playing cards multiply this number 8. You will find yourself only around 1,000 calories / day.

If you eat too little, insufficient food intake of calories to produce weight setting, will be harmful to health as they can get infected.

134. Do not go over abstinence

Many overweight, diabetic, on-diet people rush everything to lose weight fast. So not good! A person, may abstain excessive slump from 2-5 kg in a week. What then, if not dieting anymore, could be "enlarged" back. During abstinence, so the weight loss can cause the heart and other internal organs of the affected, the entire body is debilitated due to lack of nutrients. The atrophied muscle tissue also go and even body fat back, but it is also difficult to muscle recovery.

When fast weight loss, people often have symptoms:

- Anemia.

- The dull, sad or angry easily. '

- Hair loss.

- A headache.

- Kidney stones

- Sleepy.

- Prance

- Asthenia.

Therefore we need to know the value of the amount of food we eat every day has enough to provide us with the necessary calories or not. (See table of food value)

135. Reduce fat to keep weight

Americans typically get 40% of calories from fat comb. Thus, their body is about 10% balance. Fat is a source of calories. One such tablespoons oil to 120 calories gave me! Fat provides more. There is a convenient thing visible fats in our foods so easy to sort out if we want to. Here are some measures to reduce the amount of fat in your diet, keep the body from gaining weight:

- Cut small pieces of meat going to do the dishes.

- Replace red meat (beef, pork ...) with fish or poultry.

- Eliminate open in meat dishes.

- Use fat foods instead of regular - Example: milk fat has picked up.

- Avoid eating pastries.

- Eat breakfast with cereal instead of eggs and meat.

- Limit snacks, eat more, such as cakes or crunchy fried potatoes.

- Use soy yogurt mu- instead carved and fever and contact naise Mayon - chain.

- Limit your intake of butter and fries.

136. Drinking water to burn fat

Drink water to lose weight? Yes. Adults can drink 6-8 glasses of water every day is full (8-ounce glasses ..... per 220g). Why drink more water can help weight loss?

- As well drinks stay full and not want to eat anymore.

- Water helps your body digest the fat away.

- Water also helps the body fight constipation.

Here are some ways to drink a lot of water without fear:

- For a slice of lemon or orange slices in water

- Drinking fizzy water with a little more squeezed juice for a sweet savor.

- Drinking fizzy fruit juice (essentially sugar water with added flavoring).

- Pour water into the cup to find beautiful eyes.

- Those at halftime, drinking water is considered a natural job for relaxation.

137. Select the appropriate dish

There are many foods providing calories, low-calorie dishes. If you're obese, of course, should choose foods low in calories, it does offer more. But also need to know some dishes a meal an.Sau contribution here is an example of the 3 types of meals a day.

138. Purchasing something at the supermarket?

What to buy food every day so that people do not retain more fat? Prior to the supermarket, where to buy the necessities, you should:

- The first will buy the foods that do not have or was eliminate fat already. Only buy enough.

- Determined not to zone candy, cake, jam unnecessary.

- Go shopping after eating it at home. Do not go shopping when you are hungry because when food prone attractive delicious things not conducive to keeping the weight did not increase.

- Choose foods and fresh vegetables rather than ready-made foods.

- Do not buy the cakes too many nutrients.

139. When you do not eat at home

You don't often eat at home. Sometimes you need to eat, there are also fun places to take wedding invite friends. In such conditions, how to keep your diet daily followed? Please pay attention to the following tips:

- If you eat, you will choose the store has many items to yourself can choose. When looking at the food table, choose low-fat foods and provide few calories.

- Avoid the shops full of food that you like.

- Ask the waiter put the disc disk butter and bread - arbitrarily placed on the table.

- Refusal of fries and fried desserts including whether such items are included in cash and all meals.

- We should call the non-soaked barbecue dishes like butter and soap - do not mix salad oil, breads often.

- If the meat more power at home, you just cut the surplus, so to parties before eating.

- If there delicious bread, you can wrap to the breakfast in the morning. Try not to eat.

- It is possible to eat a meal with you.

- We should call each dish to order is the amount of food. Do not eat the meal of the store, prone to overeating.

When you're invited to a party or an organization fun style self-service meal, what to do?

- Go to the table and the dishes presented his decision will only eat certain foods.

- If anyone serves, he had only taken the intended food dishes.

- If possible, ask the landlord for his small vegetable dishes instead of meat dishes; no fat foods and low calorie.

- Avoid sitting near the pastries.

- You can be honest with an employer, you have to diet.

- Choose mineral water instead of wine, or drink interspersed.

- Pay attention to talk with friends rather than just paying attention to eating.

140. What to eat in large holidays?

Summer vacation holidays is great. All occasions can lead to more partying. Are you afraid your diet plan is broken or not?

- You think back to the last years of the Thanksgiving holiday, June 4, Christmas and so on ... you usually eat, not to eat too much self-restraint this year before the item.

- You remember his health status was, after that meal? How blood pressure? Having seen people uncomfortable? From there, you go to that decision how to eat during the holidays this year.

- Do not let yourself be swept under the continuous fun: this house a glass of wine, a glass and add the other house a pastry. Replace with glass of mineral water glass.

- If someone invites you to eat at home, whispered to his friend for his special diet: no fat dishes.

- Tell yourself, the holiday is mainly to meet relatives and friends. The food is secondary.

141. Choose available dishes under 100 cal.

The convenience food is available for everyone. But for those who want to keep some weight or lose weight, need to know how to choose. These foods give us most is the low-calorie dishes with our best wishes.

142. How to not think about the biscuit box?

Biscuit box in the refrigerator or in the cabinet often tempt us. How to not think about them? If you suddenly think of it, let's think of things to do to forget about them, like:

- Bring a book to read

- Call her what they ask away

- Calls to you Tom discusses the practice together so

- Manicure, pedicure and more.

143. The effect of exercise on weight loss

Many people ask the question:

Q - Exercise makes me eat better. So will increase the weight?

Dap- true that exercise makes you eat more delicious.

But, the energy consumption for greater energy exercise obtained by eating. Results: The number of calories than the calorie expenditure minimized.

Q - For weight loss, take time to practice every day?

- Just 3 times per week. 20-minute exercise sessions but if enough 45-minute episode will be better.

If you are a daily walk 30 minutes each day will help you kick was 7,5kg per year.

Q - Sweating more, faster weight loss?

Not true. Sweating so much will be risky, you should not wear more clothes when training.

Q - Aerobics any effect on weight loss?

- Aerobics including cycling, walking, swimming, affects the metabolism in the body. The impact that lasts from 4-8 hours after cessation of training. Therefore, it is good for weight loss.

144. Coordinate the two problems

To lose weight, diet is not enough. Must cooperate with the exercise again. The following is a typical number of calories consumed energy is through exercise and activity type, ask your doctor and yourself whether to join this kind of activity?

145. Effects of eating places on eating

Many people eat when they watch television, or read a book, talk to your uncontrolled eating his food intake. Therefore should:

- You must always remember that they are eating and dietary

- Eat in the eating rooms on time

- Do not do anything else while eating

- When attending the festival, focus attention on the main friends eat, drink is secondary.

- Turn off the TV smaller and music - of the program to the advertising section.

146. Diary on meals

Many people like to write a diary about their feelings every day. You can also write so with the purpose of contributing to the weight loss as follows:

- You eat when?

- There was nothing to eat, how much?

- Eat alone or with someone?

- Have you chosen what?

- After a week, you can read his diary and self-feeding so your comment will be thinner or fatter, then set out for eating expected next week.

147. Wasted exercises

Practice often generate results. But there will be no results for one kind of practice. That is the kind of exercise in thought, only in the desire, such as:

- I'll definitely be thinner.

- Being not skinny is doomed.

- It is enough to walk round

- I'll climb over walls

- I'll be picking strawberries

148. Be patient

If you stand on the scales every day, you will be discouraged, because:

- Normally, every week we lost at most only 900g. Should more than 100g daily volume for the needle does not move the needle face how much.

- 70% of our body is liquid. Many times my weight increased during the day because of drinking water,

- Does not reflect the change of the muscles and tissues.

- The weight is not as important issues you have to keep yourself in eating or not? Such dietary needs became routine for you yet?

If you are familiar with the diet, you will lose weight certain.

149. How to help young children to lose weight?

Many children of 13-15 years old were obese. How to help them lose weight. There are two problems: eating abstinence and help the children psychologically.

In doing so, pay attention to the following points:

- There is movement in family practice. For example, organizations for both biking, camping.

- In families with routine removal of fat from food.

- Everyone knows how to make low fat foods.

- Everyone knows how to stay healthy, protect teeth hair, skin

- Everyone has a plan to avoid being obese. Thus, the child will see their jobs as natural, just like people.

150. How to get used to eat less?

Wanting to lose weight, you have to limit eating. It is not easy. Therefore you must have ways, such as:

- Eat at one, as many times (5-6 times / day). eat more in the morning.

- Use small plates to share some food, though fully visible.

- Break the bread into small pieces.

- Each time cattle feed by spoon, not full of cattle.

- Chew slowly.

- Every time a party should wear tight clothing. Thus, will be afraid to eat more.

- Choose low-fat foods and plenty of water.

- After eating, brushing always. You will be afraid to eat more.

- Do not eat after dinner.

- Drink plenty of water. You'll lose your appetite for more.

- Never mind and self-promise: Today, I will eat a special meal!

151. Reward for the results

The commendation has the effect of encouraging the correct way to make results. Hence, if encouraged - either by themselves recognized the practice as the result of his weight loss, I also feel happy and more determined to continue to implement the intentions outlined.

No need to wait until you've shot for a few of weight for new self-attribution. Right from the start on a diet, you can reward yourself by doing the following:

- Buy a bouquet.

- Calls for a distant friend.

- Buy a bottle of your favorite perfume.

- Take the car wash.

- Go camping, cinema.

- Writing a diary

152. Dealing with feeling frustrated

Everyone has times of being daunting. Especially those who entered the diet. When discouraged when you do not have the courage to hold it before the lure of a good food, knowing how to eat to gain weight. These should then tell myself that this is just an interim rather than permanent surrender because:

- Everyone has time to lose the control

- Take a step back can still move on

- The struggle was long his

- The retreat also has its limits, because I have to abstain from eating, but do not eat the whole bowl!

153. Avoid being dragged into a tea cup

These studies show that psychological our actions are influenced by what we think. Based on the comments above, to prevent yourself from being drawn into the cup of tea, you can perform the following steps:

- Write a few sentences on paper to remind: "We can die of heart disease", "I have more fat," "The struggle of the decline could be" I will not be free. "

- Focus on the thinking and imagining their situation in the above case, in 20 seconds.

- Write down on paper, describe your image of that moment, (make pitiful too!)

- Imagine your pictures in the above cases in 20 seconds.

Chances are the pictures that will make you more courage not to fall into the tea cup, drinking.

154. Make yourself see the need to weight loss

When you can eject the delicious disc, be cheerful and smile. Because it was a positive action and a decision full of courage, to help you achieve the goals: reduction of body weight. Put yourself in his right: this is not a joke!

When trying to accomplish weight loss, can have two attitudes: negative and positive.

Negative people think that weight loss is just a job to her tormentor. They simply underestimate their ability to try, think things difficult enough to hamper his work as acting contaminate fresh atmosphere so. The results will come when they do not have the strength to eat anymore and really afraid for my situation.

- The area of deep thinkers saw the struggle to make weight loss a chance to practice proactive, self-restraint, endurance, to improve health for myself.

Chapter 6: How to deal with stress

The death of a loved one, divorce and illness are the main culprits causing stress. Both dated minor ailments such as having to wait over the phone when people call, they are vacuuming littered apparatus downtimes, little children again slipped down etc., all things that will make her heart sorrow, contribute to the cause of stress. But, as people have no one to avoid. Like death and taxes the same. We can do to reduce the effects of stress?

155. How to cope with stress

The death of a loved one, divorce, illness are the main culprits causing stress. Both dated minor ailments such as having to wait over the phone when people call, they are vacuuming littered apparatus downtimes, little children again slipped down etc .., all things that will make her heart sorrow, contribute to the cause of stress. But, as people have no one to avoid. Like death and taxes the same.

However, we can reduce the effects of stress to go by:

- Share your feelings with a spouse or lover, friend.

- Try to accomplish what do their job satisfaction

- Waking sleep

- Keeping health.

To avoid these phenomena are nervous tension, because of the worry, sadness after an emotional shock that, you console yourself with the following questions:

- Today I have happy news, right?

- I have to be somewhere just in time or before your appointment?

- Did you get anything right things as you want?

- Does anyone have compliments or praise me?

Finding appropriate answers, you will see the soul relieved to go.

156. Measures to reduce the effects of stress

Sometimes our stress enters quietly, very quietly. But the majority of cases, it came unexpectedly startling. In such circumstances, to reduce the shock, we should:

- Advocacy limb, take a walk around the house a few, in gardens ... let the mind calm, normal blood circulation in the veins, nervous system stabilized.

- Wash with warm water or wipe people to the muscles and nerves are relaxed.

- Confession his feelings with close friends and relatives to be comments, or share the joy or sorrow. There are people who "identify" with her, sometimes wiser and I will think of how to solve a new problem arises.

- Before the screaming, crying, because unbearable, try to count from 1 to 10.

- Pour a cup of hot tea. Drink slowly, just drinking tea breathe.

157. Rehearsal on stress

Speaker, athlete, musician and actor before the stage are the rehearsals. During training, they imagine things can happen when performed in order to find ways to cope. With stress, too. Victims may be calmer, more active if you know in advance what might happen to them when they are stressed. Contents of exercises like this:

- Close your eyes and try to make all the muscles, nerves in people sank.

- Focus on the thought for a minute, to relax and review your sense of how relaxing.

- Imagine for a minute, I'm a different person watching yourself in a relaxed state.

- Focusing the mind again to the relaxing.

- Imagine all cases that may occur when you are stressed (what happened? I feel how? Who is there then? ...)

- Imagine to his attitude at the time.

- Imagine the attitude of his relatives (spouses, friends ...) has concurred, praise, calmness and using the same time it is like.

Training twice a day so, each just 5 minutes gradually you will feel becoming tough, wise, calm down and be able to deal with any situation that occurs to me.

158. Relax muscles like?

We can set the muscles to relax each body region, from the feet to the head, according to the method of Edmund Jacobson, also known as translational relaxation techniques. You can set according to the following steps:

1. Sit on a chair and closed his eyes. Hands on a chair, hands to their backs.

2. Breathe slowly and deeply.

3. Focus the failure 'to think of a certain muscle that you can feel.

4. Ordered muscles that stretch, then sank, in 5 seconds and say that such is the body relax. Please pay attention to the feeling of relaxation that within 30 seconds, then switch to a different area of the body after doing the movements:

- Mini hands down, the new beginning at the wrist, and then to the elbow and both hands. Fists clenched and release. Relax.

- Indian back and relax on the backrests.

- Pull your tummy back and relax to soft belly back.

- Stiff jaw back and relaxing to return to normal function

- Lift the bottom leg and stretched out. Relax.

- Rolling Eyes aside and relax

- Get down to the chin touches the chest and relax.

5. Continue to breathe slowly and deeply.

6. Focusing attention on all these points to people relax and soften. Imagine yourself as dolls with rags. To head and shoulders hanging down.

7. Imagine a hot stream flow through human vitality.

8. Slowly open your eyes and see who commented how more pleasant.

Notes do not hold your breath during the learning stage and do not stress your body at the point of pain or injury.

159. Use of relaxation imagination

Imagination can turn a white cloud into red and erase the existence of stress. We have 'to use music, colors, painting in the reduction and elimination of stress.

Music - Select a music tape smoothly and find a quiet solitary place to listen to music. Imagine yourself as a part of the scenery and music. When bank notes long, you imagine yourself are spread around. While imagine, if find yourself wandering into other stories, direct your attention back to the scene and the surrounding sounds. When all tracks, compare their mental state now and before.

Colors - You imagine to 2 colors: red glare expression stress and a more subdued colors, such as pale, which shows the relaxation. Close your eyes, think of red and thinks that all his muscles are being stretched. Then you re-think of blue and imagine your muscles are being stretched. Finally you think of very pale blue color and this is regarded as a symbol of complete relaxation.

Painting - Imagine a picture of the waves beating against the rocks and the data that is considered a symbol of the tension. Then re-imagined with a peaceful scene with a small house, a few shade trees under the warm sun.

Note tracking changes in people. You will see her gentle spirit, your people and more pleasant.

160. Noting the relaxing

When nervous tension, your blood vessels to beat faster, the muscles shrink, skin, sweating, cold limbs. These phenomena may be a biological system in the body when there is stress generated each. We can based on the phenomenon to assess the state of our nerves and find ways to reduce stress in the known methods (session 158, 159). After practicing stress reduction, compare body condition before and after practice, we can self-assess their collective results more or less.

Pulse - When there is stress, rapid pulse up. Based on the pulse of the circuit before and after practice, we can infer themselves fell less stress, the body went into a state of relaxation yet.

Temperatures hand - Temperature hands can tell us neurological status because of your hands as warm demonstrate relaxation of the higher body.

Looking at the face - you try looking in the mirror and look closely at his face. Red eyes, puffy face Híp, look tired, lips curled, stiff jaw ... prove you are in a state of stress. Try relaxation. Then look at yourself, you will see the faces have changed.

161. Method actively relax

Just think of language fingernails scraped across a blackboard, or when you bite into a lemon small enough to shudder. Such a thought can cause us feel.

We can use the method of "self-reflection" to relieve the tension of the muscles in the chronic headaches. For example, you use a number of sayings, repeated in order to make yourselves feel, in the limbs or the cozy feeling. The feelings that attracted his attention to reduce stress and relax nerves.

Here is an example of multiple steps:

1. Choose a quiet place. Turning off the lights to dim light only. Wear warm clothes, sitting relaxed in a recliner and closed his eyes.

2. Start talking about your hand. If you are right-handed, then talk about the right hand front, left-handed, the left hand before talking about such as:

- The arm weighs too (mentioned 3 times)

- Feet weighs too (3 times)

- Both feet too heavy and my hands (3 times)

To easily imagine, may be forced into the hands, feet, a small object, slightly heavier.

3. The following are methods create a warm feeling by saying:

- My hands warm too (each hand, say 3 times)

- My feet warm too (each leg, say 3 times)

- Hands, my feet warm too (mentioned 3 times. For ease of imagination can soak hands and feet in hot water, or sit sun).

Note: Those who are nervous or cure treatment with medication, should consult a physician before using this method.

162. Soak in water and let the body float

Imagine yourself floating in warm water, in a dark place, with no light. Around completely silent except for a voice of their own breathing. You absolutely nothing to stress identifier. All EAC flesh in the person you are in a state of maximum relaxation, mental clarity.

That is the method used to - like - value - whether in a narrow environment, also called immersion method - who drop - floating effect makes your heart and lungs work slowdown, floppy muscles, all feel tension because of stress disappear.

To get that state, where treatment with the above method, we build the salt water tank, just for a person lying on. The salinity of the water, making it easy to float. I lie in pools of water, to celebrities and imagine lying on a mattress miracle.

In a dark room without noise, or there may be a slight soft music of their favorite songs.

Each time soaking - people - celebrities such Tha- long distance for one hour. When referring to step out of the water, I feel people cheery stress because stress reduced or disappear.

This method has many advantages:

- Listening to music while soaking - people - drop - minded celebrities such as gentle.

- The floating on warm water conditioning effects in blood vessels.

- Water splash on people doing the joints pain, people from aches, nausea for no more pills.

Care with: This method is suitable for everyone.

People who are nervous therapist should talk to your doctor before using this method.

163. Do not be afraid to cry

When suddenly crying for happiness, crying because of an infinite sadness or for any emotional reasons, the tears will calm your emotions, reducing the intensity of stress. Thus, it is beneficial to health.

Scientists from the University of Minnesota have isolated Hoe 2 important components in tears, leucine enkephalin and substance prolacitin substances. The two substances are present only when we cry because emotions. The other causes of watery eyes - as when we peel onions, a little practice such as burning eyes - no two chemicals in tears. Leucine enkephalin substance is a substance secreted by the brain's response secrete substances "consolation" This is a job with health benefits. William Frey, a biochemist studying also said that tears wash away the harmful substances accumulate in some points of the body, in times of stress.

In such context, any time we feel the need to cry, do not be afraid. Let the tears flowed. After crying, people find greater peace gloating.

Men often compressed emotions to show that he is tough guy. They rarely cry for women, Maybe so, but every time what events emotional impact, the man was dispatched easily fall sick and beaten most regulations.

164. The effect of laughter

From an immemorial time, people have known that smile has very good influence on the body. Greek people believe that laughter keeps a significant role in restoring the health of the patient. These studies have demonstrated today, when people laugh better blood circulation, lowered blood pressure, digestion and brain easily endorphins secreted analgesic effect. Therefore, not only wanted to joke that the other doctors have told patients: "Take two aspirin and think this a funny story to tell me at the time to visit sick tomorrow."

To preserve the health and laughter relaxed, do the following things:

- Imagine you are looking through the lens of a video camera is recording the activities of many people. Thus, sight and his thoughts about everything that happened, will be broader and more open.

- Every day, take the time to read or listen to stories laugh.

- Do not just smile. Should laugh for real into gloating.

- When you encounter a shopkeeper selling seems sedate face or a person who is raising her arms to carry a heavy cargo, imagine them wearing only an underwear with embroidery for women.

- When meetings, chat, keep cheerful attitude. Sometimes witty, humorous blow to swap stories about work to help you come up with ideas lucid communication hub and tighten the friendship.

- In trade, laughter can help you profit. That is the secret of "smile out of money".

- Do not be afraid to laugh alone and took to himself.

- Remember, people are living longer smiling.

165. Accepting the criticism

You can be easily angry with others' criticism? If you have any comments you feel difficult to understand well, please feel calmly brushed it aside to ponder his next.

You turn on the oven because of criticism over how? There are odd words to touch her like he's so fat, she slowly bubbling bubbling, booming voice vv..thuc out just words reflect truth outwardly unimportant as the words touched their self-esteem.

But, if you are those who have confidence in yourself, believe in your nature, sooner or later, those words are untrue to you will melt like soap bubbles alone, nothing worth the throne.

However, it was found that even with one of the other criticisms are accurate. Having thus, we will repair our weaknesses. And the other words? To know that you need to pay attention to it or not, ask yourself board:

- Criticism of the other has not? There is no discernable point or not?

- I have one criticism of this or not?

- The critics say this has to understand the implications and effects of that word or not? (If the school itself is not likely to understand, then we should ignore).

- Are criticisms for me or not? Or is it just generalities himself again and grabbed his startled?

- Criticism based on views that differ from my opinion? (If there are free response).

If you think that criticism correctly, so courageously taken up, if small steps for-one. Doing so only in their favor.

166. Cut off the stressful thoughts

If you are under stress by a single idea, try to cut off that thought away. For example, someone comments on something you do wonder if you stab the hour, cannot concentrate on anything else. So how do you have? Follow those steps:

1. Find ways to deceive the thoughts about it aside.

2. Close your eyes and focus attention on the eyes closed.

3. Count to three.

4. Shout "Stop!" (If there are more people around, no means loud, think about the sea with "Stop!", or imagine a traffic light suddenly turned red lights and the words "Stop!"

5. If the mind is still thinking about the old, counting to five.

6. Open your eyes, continue to work normally.

You can use this method every time a job or want to forget what a haunting image makes you tired and you do not focus on other work.

167. Avoid anxiety over 5 stages

Every day there are 13 million Americans who often seem as having worried pensive face. The report by the Institute of Mental Health said, apparently worried such a negative impact on health.

So people often worry about what? Often about what might happen in the future.

According to Thomas Borkovec psychologist at the University of Pennsylvania, who is also related to their jobs worry, but should limit them in certain period. To reduce anxiety, one should follow the following 5 steps:

1 Know the signs before we worry as: can not concentrate, sweating hands, felt like objects fall on the abdomen.

2. To permanently half hours every day to take care to everything.

3. Write down your issues are concerned.

4. Resolve or proposed measures to address these issues during the half hour was specified.

5. In addition to the time out, determined not to think about that problem anymore. If the mind is also concerns about things that look for something to do to forget about it or use methods such as cutting off thinking at all 166.

168. Do not become workaholic

Many of people demand too much, work too much and are always in a hurry, busy life, want to complete a lot of works in the shortest time. Such people, unavoidable stress. Here are the steps to slow down its work, limiting their workaholic:

- On what date no one, no work left to do right when working hours, leave a wristwatch to stay home.

- Each time only do one thing only. For example, do not just read while listening to the phone reports.

- Try to speak slowly. When other people are saying, and I do not fully understand the people to speak, then do not interrupt.

- Go slow and steady steps. Do not go half and half sensitivity.

- When one acquaintance should look to see who it is

- Greet and smiled at them. Do not walk and think.

- Driving under the correct speed or permitted.

- When waiting for the phone, or a phone call to someone, try not to fidget.

- Between the meetings will take time 15 minutes break for mind relaxation.

- Every day should be spent resting at a certain time. Determined not to do something in the meantime.

- Spend more time to observe the surroundings, identify the good, the beautiful scenery around me.

169. Use of time

We cannot extend, cannot borrow, cannot sell time and also cannot stop it. Everyone has 24 hours a day, 7 days a week. But there are people who know how to use time effectively than others. Want to be like that, so how?

- Make an inventory of all the work - you go into a statistics kind of work: work that you need to do first, what to do second. Thus, you will have an overview about his work and imagine what they must do to decide what matters.

Ratings jobs - jobs should be classified as type A (to be done immediately, as soon as possible); Type B (not urgent anymore) and Class C (can do in the long term ...)

- Avoid overlapping jobs - Remember that the ability of each person are limited, time, too. Therefore, to identify themselves only solve 'anything in days.

- Distinguish the daily chores and lucrative job: daily chores, such as call - the phone; arranged books and papers. These things can make progress also. The work related to the production, co lucrative purposes, to settle a definitive step. If possible, should do much more lucrative job as a chore.

- Think about the time passed in vain for the day. It's time to go sit chatting or calling ca la dating or meeting is not necessary. Must shorten this time again.

- Cannot be disturbed - should have the attitude to let people know what their spare time to time you do not want to be disturbed. But then, close the office door and let others answer his phone instead.

- Utilize your time wisely see the day. In a day, there is time to feel the most comfortable person. Should list the important work to address at that time.

- Do not be too perfectionist - should do their best, but also remember that nothing is completely without shortcomings. If left too much effort to want to be able to do something for the complete truth clearly, will lose futile and wasted time.

- Avoid hesitated, not definitive - If you find yourself hesitating do not believe in, whether it results or not, ask yourself: "Why not use this time to do other more profitable?"

170. Do not work constantly

People are working constantly throughout the day. Doing so will produce stress. With these people, have time off and outdoors are essential. Making such continual can:

- Obtain few results.

- Make you ignore family and those who are around you.

Irrespective of what is important, it does not need.

Often when there is an unusual matter what happens, who work tirelessly type who feel the slowest. Because such work, mind crashing out "dazed" and.

- Ask the wife (husband) or your friends to know you're the type that the case? If you answered 'yes', then here are a few' keeper drugs "that you can use:

- Reduce the number of hours you usually work every day down. Imagine working weekdays as weekend days. Rather an important work by Class B Class A as working in the maintenance program of the day.

- Record in the work program of the day both time and breaks as well as a job here.

- Take time for physical activity: exercise, walking or participating in the games without thinking.

- During the meal, do not talk about work.

- During the holiday period, select the activity opposed to paperwork, the holidays should go camping, outdoor bike, to visit relatives. The work day often requires you to calculate, think the holidays, you can sew or knit etc.

Should choose fun activities the whole family can participate.

- When not working, do not feel like I was guilty.

171. What to do with traffic congestion?

Vehicles block the road. The bad weather. Last week, you have to go slow to 3 times. Therefore, in the car, but as half a burning heart.

To avoid such circumstances on, what should you do?

- Before going to work, should listen to the radio announcement to know there is traffic congestion phenomenon in any way?

- When traveling, as avoid the main road, but winter, as well.

- Go to work 10 to 15 minutes earlier than the time to prevent traffic jams.

- View a map to remember the small road, on the way his side can use, when the main road is blocked.

If you have a room far away, but you still do not get rid of traffic jams, not because of that that makes her nervous stress, useless. Here are a few tips:

- Do not think of the wheel is standing still.

- Take a few slow, deep breaths.

- Do not blame those things that cannot be changed, for example: in a bad driver, in his number of black.

- Note Ad words on the radio to forget the existing circumstances.

- Listen happy music tapes, stories or lessons about autonomy.

- Get out a pen and paper to record their intentions to carry out within days, the list of things I need to buy toys and more.

Those measures, not only do you lose time in vain help but cheer you at the car spirit continues to run, when the road was all blocked.

172. Stay calm when there are events

According to the Institute of Psychiatry, then within 6 months, up to 30 million Americans have to deal with an event in their lives, such as job loss, bereavement, illness, accident, emotional trouble.

The grief caused by those events even be multiplied, depending on the feelings and reactions of each person, leading to a state of stress as a destiny. In fact, we can use a number of measures to lessen the impact of those events on the spirit and our health, such as:

Think of the future is key. "After the rain comes the sun", when people look at things with the eyes of optimism, the unfortunate things happen will also go down effects.

- Application of the methods known to relax the body at the beginning of this chapter.

- So said the incident objectively.

Avoid cultural importance, as to talk to. While recounts should not be used as way of saying: "always" "never seen so", "cannot withstand truth"

- Solve work slowly, step by step. Does not require her to how to break away from the new situation occurs.

- Do not lower yourself before difficulties, but should recognize the help of everyone. Love, friendship, social assistance are very precious resource for your relay overcome stress during this time.

- Remember, not alone such circumstances you encounter. Many others have gone through situations like that, so they have a lot of experience to help you overcome.

173. Holding anger

Not only the boss but also the director, the head of the agency can have irritability. All employees, from construction worker, who sat at his desk, housewives, until a few artists are also like that.

Generally, those who are anxious to complete their work, or sometimes feel too tired because of work becomes difficult fastidious streak, or anger.

In fact, anger is not falling from the sky. It was smoldering in my heart for a long time, nourished by the warm memories from the job information failed hopes are fading, as the small flame waiting for the opportunity is flared. Therefore, it also has symptoms such as:

- Boring

- Feeling tired

- Loss of confidence

- Work is not effective.

- No enthusiasm, indifferent to everything.

Each one expressed his losing control one way: with people, face severe as sinners, while others are frowning, grumpy, aggressive work, heavy legs. They often 'do not get mistakes on his part that or blame and blame others. These things often does no good but only winds helped ease their anger flared only. To curb the temper should:

- Pay attention to the state of the body, such as insomnia, bloating and other unusual phenomena.

- Self question whether you desire something in your career and in life. Is what I wished for real or not? If not, should change or lower the target down to their level can reach.

- We should separate their personal work out.

- Sometimes, should identify themselves as left-calculated. Only a small thing also want to do a big story.

- Reduce the time to work or going to your little comfort can work. Do not let your work turned into slaves.

- Learning the mental relaxation techniques and body to avoid stress. Relaxation helps us to work easily and quickly.

- If participation exercise to be physically active, but pay attention if his career was the nature of the competition, the practice should not lose any more feeding. In such cases, only the best jogging.

174. The spirit of optimism

Turning defeat into gaining, turning risk into a garment, said to himself: "Failure is the mother of success", that is the secret of the special use of optimistic spirit to rise above every difficulty. They considered the stumbling at work are lessons to train yourself more experience. Want such possibility, we should:

- Do not walk backwards considered a failure

- Considering the fact unfortunately is an opportunity to challenge yourself

- Always ask the question: "By what I could have done this better?" instead the question: "This may lead to something bad?"

- To consider the difficult step is a chance to rest, convalescence before entering new fighting game.

- Always on the attack. In match racing talent, if we cannot control, you control your opponent is yourself. Keeping the initiative is to capture more wins.

- Do not overpower others and yourself.

- It should set out the objectives widely. Do not just look at things is, however within a day.

175. Prevent tension in the family

Causes of stress sometimes start right at home. Nobody can do anything for the good, if in the family there is always change, disintegration instead of seat of the "staff" to deal with things in life.

Many social psychologists believe that the family is a unit capable of help to people who live together, are easily overcome difficult moments such as the loss of the illness.

Here are some ideas to eliminate stress from the family atmosphere, where every member of the family needs to know:

Creating conditions for everyone in the family had the opportunity to talk to each other regularly and keep the same feelings of solidarity among the members of the family.

- Keep the habits, customs and family gatherings. In this meeting, should set out the common work, the future is expected. Should avoid blaming each other, spend time solving problems peacefully conflicts. Each person should remember the family's meeting calendar for the next year to contribute their opinions to the family and relatives.

- Should pay attention to hear the opinions of others and understand public opinion, the murmur of disagreement of the children and grandchildren to discuss settlement.

- Assign general meeting dates based on anniversaries or birthdays of loved ones.

- It is thought to reflect deeply about the value of solidarity.

- Feedback for members whenever required changes as important as job loss, should change jobs or other jobs. Comforted the members when meeting events.

- They must believe in the ability and attention to the interests of each member, should not be compared, and discrimination between women and men: sons and daughters, brothers and sisters v v ... Each members, though younger and are free and have the right to decide in a certain range.

- Eliminate thoughts envy, jealousy, ethnical.

- Do not just focus on the membership status and more money.

176. Avoid stress for young people

Remember that young children are also members of the family, the children adjacent to adulthood usually have many questions, wondering what happened to the family, in society. Therefore, children need guidance and help of adults. You should:

- Have the opportunity to quiet, deserted to chat, learn about what the children questions, concerns. Stories should choose simple, easy to understand, is thicker meaning to explain their concerns.

- Ask him about the symptoms of stress that the children might have, such as sweating hands, feeling heavy hearted.

- Guidelines for the children of methods to reduce stress as:

Breathe slowly and deeply, exhale Now, imagine yourself acting out the anxiety, sorrow in her genealogy blasts into the air.

Visualize to warm scenes of the family as, that at the moment are lying comfortably in bed, was playing in the yard, sitting as the TV with the whole family, sitting neatly in his lap and so on ...

- Encourage your child deep breathing and etched into the minds of the family warm scene later to lean on images that transcend the emotions anxiety, fear, sadness whenever trouble, monitoring ash.

Chapter 7: How emotions have effect on health and vice versa

A person with a cold, arthritis or heart attack will automatically look for the rescue, ready to tell people to help themselves and if necessary, ask for permission to leave for treatment.

But when there is an emotional pain, they do not behave like that. Not everyone heard them talk, they asked for help and whether the disease has affected the health and ability to work, no one resigned because of a personal love story.

Scientists study on humans are recognized to be associated closely between psychology and physiology. Some men get sick and mentally declining, usually aged 50 or over. People alone or with emotional problems were killed, twice as many people have a happy family. A year after her husband died, 60% of the widow began a period of illness, weakness. Number of single men in the United States died prematurely before the age, level with the man died from nicotine addiction.

In this program, we will address the issues related to emotions, such as anger, jealousy, obsessed by sin, depression etc. We also seek remedies to cure mental illnesses such as music, climate and the mutual pampering spoiled.

Of course, mental illnesses can become physical illness and your ability to treat many psychological disciplines as medicine, more effective than the drugs a lot.

177. Getting over being sorrow

Sighing, sulking, muttering, screaming and throwing furniture are the expression of the heart seem bothered much longer in keeping people can be converted into a number of diseases such as a headache, rash, stomach pain or high blood pressure.

If you experience these things not pleasant, should adopt the following measures to alleviate problems troubling bout:

- When you feel her heart begin to feel unhappy to count from one to ten and breathe three, four little slow and deep.

- If you have seen sulking in picking up people who want to, you walk a few rounds until the storm subsided sad.

- Do not grumble, blame. If someone says something that you do not agree, so calm discussion, feedback.

- We should find ways to make yourself happy. If you're on a car trip, stuck because of traffic congestion, tell yourself: I cannot feel anything more be.

Honk or urge the driver will remain like that; but even more pissed off. Up to that time to listen to music, or watching a funny story.

178. Tame jealousy

When a colleague is arranged sitting on the chair that you are expecting, or has a release latch joked with someone you love, you feel a little angry, it is something natural. But if you are so miserable because of jealousy that you get the real skinny, it is not recommended.

Jealousy often arise when a person other than his or scaring people consume something or someone they are also preferred. Jealousy was born skeptical.

To tame or reduce jealousy, should:

- Recognize that I am jealous. Self knows this also helps you to cope more sober towards himself.

- When you see other people succeed, so happy for it and use it as a mirror to try to complete its work.

- Always keep your good nature.

Remember, jealousy may terminate friendship or love burgeoning. If you think that in his heart thoughts suspect someone you love (husband and wife), so think about what can make your mind towards other work: e.g. expected revised his apartment in . It should not take long to turn the suspect asked her about it.

179. Elimination of inferiority

It is a mistake when feeling about ourselves and having followed wishes than is supposed to do for others. Many people may have feelings for their jobs find themselves always felt wrong and at fault to remove the inferiority complex which:

- Do not always do the will of others. Must be confident, know your abilities, your job goal.

- Do not always show courtesy and calm.

If sometimes you're too impatient, irritable, it is normal and is not necessary to regret it.

- Do not take time to accuse his own works. If you consider what is wrong, it should draw experience from catching the next time and think how correct way for good.

- Should be satisfied with his part finished better than yourselves restless with his unfinished section.

180. Interruption of a nervous breakdown

The changes in life such as divorce, having relatives lost, losing jobs can make us collapsed. Especially it can imagine gear towards affordability and make us worried and sick again. But sometimes, the mental breakdown seems to be not definitive. Yet, we still feel:

- Sad and empty.

- The feeling alone, frustrated, guilty remorse.

- Not keen on the job, including sexual activity.

- Sleep does not sleep, tossing and turning.

- Feeling no enthusiasm.

- Difficulty concentrating and did not want to decide anything.

- There are symptoms such as the headaches, digestive disorders medication not cured.

To cut off this phenomenon, should take the following measures:

- Replacement head pessimistic thoughts with positive thoughts.

- Relations with the optimists, are intoxicated with life, with work. They will get you excited over.

- Do not just think about yourself. Should do something to help others.

- Participating in daily exercise, or at least as walking the dog. Better, cycling, playing tennis went shopping for furniture.

- Do something different from the usual, such as travel to a place I have not been to either go to eat at a new restaurant.

- It is expected to do a job there, without hardly just fun.

If feelings of depression, mental breakdown was extended to three weeks, should consult their doctor to know what disease, tell your doctor or hearing you have used drugs or are using to see if it is reaction to the drug or not.

181. How to avoid disappointment after the holidays

- After the holidays including Christmas Day, many people are not happy but frustrated and sad. Why so? Maybe because of the following reasons:

- Not having enough relatives. There are people in far not the family.

- Remembering deceased relatives.

- Lack of money.

- Too tired for work and holiday rituals.

- Expect more noble things in the holidays.

For the following public holidays without feeling disillusioned, depressed, you should apply the following measures:

- Preparation before the job to stay up to date, not been too busy.

- Expected written invitations or special confectionery for those of earlier ones.

- Do not drink alcohol because alcohol will cause you feeling tired, pessimistic the next day.

- Do not place too high expectations for the holidays such as confectionery must fully and work to decorate the house is beautiful, the people enough who face no shortage etc ...

- No detail is too likely.

- If you see the organization according to the rules, the old routines too restrictive in nature should be left to follow the new rules.

- If you want to get yourself comfortable alone in the holidays, do not wait for someone invited her to attend the fun anywhere, and do not invite anyone or appointment.

182. Avoid the sad winter storm

November, along with the return of winter, many people find heavy heart melancholy. The feeling that lasts throughout the season and just melts away as next spring. Scientists call this phenomenon is the spirit of seasonal disorder.

Light and temperature have profound influence trite phenomenon. The sun's rays stimulate the brain to secrete chemicals that enhances the dynamics of the body. There are about 5% of people in humanity felt sad when the time has light of a shorter day. We can use fluorescent light, replacing sunlight to cure melancholy of winter.

If in the winter, you naturally feel sad - sadness inorganic, should:

- Go outside as much as possible, good morning than the afternoon.

- As long as there bright outdoors, expand the veil door.

- The overcast cloudy day, so turn on the lights in the house.

Do not sit alone daydreaming. Please visit friends, go to a museum, go see the exhibition and more.

- You can take a break in the winter instead of summer vacation.

183. How to deal with sadness

After the unhappy events such as the death of a loved one, divorce, unemployment and sickness usually persistent grief. Sometimes people forget that it went great, but then the pain came back with a head full of new phase as a sudden illness and became a dull pain inside. We want to deny reality but is not, and must accept it as the truth.

To sustain this part grief, you can follow some of the following measures:

- Do not hide your feelings and also not shy expressed those feelings.

- Friends and family members who are willing to sympathize and share the pain with you.

- Write a diary about the incident as well as calming somewhat grief. It should be written in the expected direction with the brighter days ahead.

- Do not take alcohol and food to forget sorrow.

- Keep eating in moderation, nutrients added.

- Notice of rest and convalescence light exercise to stay healthy during this time.

- Avoid being alone during the holidays or birthdays.

- While not all sadness in my heart, then their spirit is not yet clear. Therefore, should not decide what is important during this time.

- The business during this period is often not smooth. May have to accept a setback.

- If you feel tired, do not take on the job, need to ask someone for help or temporarily replaced to solve the task.

184. Learn about the obsession

Before tooth extraction or when driving in heavy rain, thunder rumble, it is felt like when we had to stay home alone in the childhood. The feeling of fear only happen in a short time and then off. But many people have the fear response nature body, prolong life, and in interaction with the spirit, both physiological impact as strong heartbeat, sweating, vomiting, choking and more when the victim fainted: fear has become a frequent obsession directly available in person, such as:

Afraid to look down deep (it is impossible to drive on mountain roads in the edge region).

- Fear of looking into the distance widely;

- Fear of cats, afraid of mice;

- Afraid of blood.

- Afraid of the dark.

These are emotions related to psychological problems of each person. By practice and treatment by a psychologist, 80% of people with such diseases can from.

185. The impact of music on humans

Everyone felt rustling sea waves that affect nerve as sedative. Many doctors' extractions twist to soft music in the waiting room for patients feeling less anxious.

Many places in the hospital, people use cassettes with birdsong. In the large pavilion of the supermarket, the music sometimes forget to do the time, do not want to. The soft music, slow heartbeat may slow down and blood pressure reducing effect of the fruit with intense music, fast and turn up.

You can make an impact on your music as follows:

- To relax, you should choose which works with at the climax as

"The section G Major for strings grams" of Bach; "The music chasing each gram Ré" by Pachelbel; 'Concerto for Cello grams Ré "by Haydn;" moonlight "by Debussy and more ...

- The music fast, high can pull you from the state of melancholy, rueful.

- The music has the same speed smooth beats of the heart alone make small children cry.

- To stimulate employees to work with the results, use simple tunes, popular songs.

Also recommend changing rhythms and music from time to time: the morning should use funny songs, before lunch, jerky gestures, firing in the afternoon, the quiet music.

186. What is the benefit of having a pet?

Who does not want to laugh when looking at the dogs or two cats playing with each other? Many Americans consider dogs, pet cats as friends can share feelings with people at the happy, sad, or lonely, because:

- They make us cherish attitude, care.

- They seem to believe in our care.

- We get our feelings without hesitation, thinking.

- We make those who are lonely, feel assured that comfort of the elderly. In addition to dogs and cats, the activities of the swim around the aquarium can make people forget worries, sadness and reduce blood pressure for people with the disease.

Many families feel more intertwined, cozy family atmosphere because the presence of a dog.

187. Who can easily catch cancer?

Currently, cancer is still one of the most formidable disease to humans, because the scientists have not yet been fully defined causes.

Is it because of the smoke, breathing inhaling toxins or contaminated? They also ask the question: why people smoke, the lung cancer, but other people do not smoke like that again?

Many researchers say that the streak, the behavior of each person has more or less influence to the disease.

- There are passive, indifferent to everything.

- Or her feelings compression, not want to express out.

- To the anger, hatred smoldering in person.

- When there are events not to occur, often self-isolation does not want the help or comfort of others.

- Over the strenuous or emotional disturbance during adolescence.

When people have such streak on cancer, they often accept their fate unfortunately easily and death to them and very quickly. An explanation of the relationship between the streak and susceptible, the doctors said that positive streak, preferred activities, openness of the phenomenon of human stimulation, hormone secreted by the side effects body against the disease. Even the person with cancer, but the body was fighting against the disease in the long term are often those who work, or ask, ask of other people, open and easy to express feelings mine.

188. How to detect and prevent suicidal status quo

If someone knows your talking suicidal intentions, you should not despise and ignore. The familiar saying of suicidal despondent man is usually:

"The things that no longer mean anything to me anymore." "I've had enough of this life time ago", or more clearly, "I just want to die?"

The despondent man also had the attitude:

Such as what is important, no hope of any one thing, do not need any help.

- Sleep is restless.

- At the ability to think, concentrate, decided something.

- Standing alone, do not want to interact with others.

- For all his personal belongings.

To prevent and avoid the phenomenon of suicide, should not:

- Ignoring suicidal threats.

- Concealing suicidal idea of someone

- Challenge who intend suicidal.

- To the person with suicidal intentions alone. Candle:

- Find info intentions who have this intention, and whether they have guns or "drugs" anything?

- Should contact friends, family doctor to give advice.

- Tell the weary idea that many people already know their intentions and ready to help them overcome difficulties in employment, life.

They are not to despair as they thought. - Encourage them to work again and engage in collective action, training and entertainment along with everyone.

189. When to seek help of experts?

Sometimes you have to work private or professional nature that they cannot solve someone help, there must be close friends, but they are not always near him. Furthermore, their ability to make anything more without having any conversation with you is also revealed.

In that case, you need to mentors, experts, who specialize in the issues that you are entanglements. They will help you to point you the way to go so you can get the job resolution. When you need the help of professionals? That's when you have:

- The prolonged mental decline.

- The change in mood.

- Being psychosis of fear or anxiety.

- There is grief and tormented past that has now returned.

- Drinking too much alcohol, or drug abuse.

- Have digestive disorders (vomiting after eating).

- Obsessed with the image or the incident was over, both during work.

- New know-threatening illness or debilitating health.

These professionals can help you efficiently when you lose a job, recently divorced, have relatives who died or have other trouble.

People who have hallucinations, like hearing voices and strange sounds, meant to commit suicide, not their autonomy, their fear may have illegal actions etc. Are needed to right the heart specialist Management for help.

190. Which advisers should be chosen?

For example, you are having trouble emotionally such as anxiety, anger, grief, regret, you should have advisers who counseled. There are two issues to consider when selecting their advice: it is the expertise of the adviser and the acquaintance between you and advisers like? "The research says about this: you know or are not familiar with or do not have feelings for advisers unconnected with the guidelines and methods that mentor used to solve the problem you are obstacles.

Should be based the following criteria to select their mentors and act as follows:

Tell your summarized issues and problems and ask advisers have solved problems similar or not?

- Talk to your counselor wants help and how he will use what methods to solve effectively.

- Do you find yourself believing in the experience of the adviser does not?

- Ask advice about the time needed to solve this problem. Nor should the request must be completed in a short time or the timing of the work. Often, sometimes have a new monthly resolved.

- Find out the cost of this, you get the Department of Insurance does not spend?

- If you want advice about marriage or about sexual issues, should give the lover or wife (husband) go.

Chapter 8: How to overcome an addiction

Each person being addicted to tobacco, alcohol, drugs has different reasons: to enjoy extreme stimulation, escape the boredom of everyday life to make yourself seem more elegant people etc. Then when feeling vibrations, the pride tinged with joy has passed, they are the only body aches, as an objective look lifeless pancreas. Particularly cigarette smoke was put 390,000 Americans each year across the world, earlier than their age. Yet still another 50 million people continue to smoke. It's crazy, we even do not mention that 10% of Americans drink.

Alcohol has many broken families, many who lost their jobs in the health situation of collapse. Also to mention the many other drugs that had earlier been unknown as marijuana, cocaine and heroin Both hypnotics and sedatives medications that people take too much longer.

The chapter recently introduced to you the measures to be able to keep us from getting into toxic substances or help the addicts get rid of dark circles there.

191. You are a slave of addiction or not?

The culprit of the addiction to tobacco is nicotine. A tobacco researcher said: "If there is no nicotine cigarette smoking is also nothing more than blowing bubbles games".

There are people sensitive to nicotine than others, so the more addictive. The test questions in the table below will be of you know I got my leg into the trap of nicotine to the extent then, was a slave of it or not?

192. Test lungs by matchstick

In the birthday, do you feel blowing out the candle is a difficult thing? If so, you are smokers, the lung has been hurt because of smoke.

Test your lung capacity by the following steps:

1. Mark a match. When the flames are burning, not shaken again, to how his mouth 15 cm.

2. Inhale and breathed air into the (mouth open, not bunched up). Can be breathed repeatedly.

3. If the flame is not, you've been smoke lung damage and should go to the doctor.

193. Seven responses

Knowing smoking is harmful, but addicts often pointed to several reasons for marshal. The following are the common reasons and yet comment.

1. If I quit smoking, I will obese to lose!

In fact, quitting is not fat, but because eating more than before. If you want to keep the weight or lose weight, you can participate in daily exercise and attention fat diet, avoid junk food, in addition to meals.

2. I see many people smoking and still healthy!

Small portions, or less sick time. But there are things you definitely do not in some people that.

3. Tobacco cannot "lower" I'm not? Whatever you cannot die of tobacco but you will suffer from certain diseases such as: difficulty breathing, cough, hypertension, cardiovascular disease ... is diseases that doctors will force you to stop smoking. So why do not you quit before?

4. Cigarettes make me relax.

Nicotine is a stimulant nervous and makes the adrenal glands secrete adrenaline. Adrenaline is a hormone with militant or "fiery" nature do not relax anywhere.

5. I've tried to quit smoking without any food 12th losing 12 or 17 is just a number. Not yet, continue until the withdrawal is. Those who are drug withdrawal are also enduring spirit and determination so!

6. Quitting is so hard!

You can see people upset. No one died of smoking cessation at all. You should believe that their withdrawal be!

7. Cannot imagine life without drugs?

When born, you did not know smoking is. Smoking is a habit only. Therefore, when not smoking, then you've seen life after quitting happy, life is still fun.

194. Spending on tobacco

Can you believe how much smokers have spent on smoking?

In addition to the money spent on the above, there should be including additional clause:

- Payments for matches, lighters.

- Clothing, carpets ... speckled burnt because cigarette butts.

- Cash rated cement floor.

- Lotions, toothpastes, dental mouthwash for smokers.

- On medical leave

- Dental treatment medications

- Spending on health insurance.

Smokers have to spend more of the preceding paragraphs, the average annual distance of 700 dollars (USD)

195. Quitting? Nothing is difficult!

Writer Mark Twain said:

"You want to quit smoking, huh? What's difficult, I know ... So the rule I've ever sucked a hundred times before that?" Hearing that, the withdrawal easy or difficult? Mainly before withdrawal, you must carefully prepare both physically and mentally for themselves and believe that I can rule it!

Here is the step by step of the 3 phases smoking cessation.

196. Candy of nicotine to get over addiction

Though it is late, it is still better! It was only in 1988, through interviews of 2,000 scientists, it has been officially recognized: smoking is harmful to health; the phenomenon is caused by tobacco addiction nicotine. Therefore, want to detox, not to ignore the smoking habits but also to think about the measures that the body has the ability to fast, is not exposed to this material again.

One measure is the researchers applied during body detox remain exposed to nicotine, but in small doses. So will not cause much discomfort for the ruler. The doctor will give the detoxification suck or chew the candies gum that contains nicotine.

Dose candy also lessened. Thus the ruler smoking will avoid the frequent phenomenon in the absence of drugs, such as nausea, ourselves, irritability, sleeplessness, having a headache and so on.

If you want to quit smoking, should follow the following:

- DIY test under article 191. If your total score of 7 or higher, you have to govern according to the method outlined.

- Talk with your doctor your intention to quit smoking, to the doctor's suggestions if you are pregnant women should not eat this candy. Those with heart disease and high blood pressure, too.

- When using the gum, must comply with the instructions of the doctor or the instructions on how to package candy.

Want to quit smoking with the result, should coordinate the use of candy with smoking cessation measures Article 195.

197. Throw away the pipe?

Smoking cigars or using the pipe after dinner is the normal habit of man. Fortunately that, from 25 years ago, many people have the habit because many of them were suffering from diseases such as cancer, larynx, throat and esophagus.

If you have moderate smokers smoking a pipe, you can also add other illnesses questions as: coughing, heart disease and lung cancer as well. As well as smoking cessation, want to quit smoking cigars or using a pipe tobacco, you also need to follow the following measures:

1. For a few days of research, pay close attention to their habits as smoking (smoking where: in the living room, the car, at work, after a meal v. V ...)

2. Every time you are about to take a cigarette, stop and delay in 1 hour. Do this for several days.

3. Limit smoking venue. Now, just in front of the doorway smoking, for example.

4. Increase the cigarette delayed from 1 hour to 2 hours.

5. While smoking, not to read, watch TV or anything else.

6. Only half of cigarette smoke, leaving the other half to go.

7. Finally, quit, do not smoke anymore.

198. Chewing nicotine is harmful?

Besides smoking, nicotine can be put on people by chewing or snuffing. Smoking, chewing, inhalation are equally harmful, for health. Example: put nicotine on people chew through the thin membrane in the mouth. The tissue exposed to nicotine in the mouth prone thickens: it is the first point of attack cancer.

Best not exposed to tobacco, regardless of any type. Here are some suggestions for you to do:

- Do not consider any position on tobacco advertising.

- If the urge to smoke, replace nicotine by chewing gum, mints or chewing dental fragrance.

- Participation in sports activities.

- Self reward yourself after a day not exposed to tobacco

199. Please help others quit smoking

Berate, ridicule, scolding them is not a good method to get rid of smoking addiction.

If you want to help someone quit smoking, should:

- Tell them ready for their help more effort, determination to quit. Separate means they must have the will to quit, his only encourage it.

They help the family household as childcare, household kitchen while they quit.

- Do you have suggestions and comments, not to steer more to do this, to do that. Let the smoking cessation initiative in his work.

- Encourage them to keep your spirits high. Although annoyed by being so stubborn ruler.

200. Alcohol drinking in moderation

We have not discussed about the issue whether we should drink or not, we just only talked about: people need to know their body, how much alcohol they can tolerate. The table "effect of alcohol on the body" will show you clearly the mental state, gestures, our actions depend on the concentration of alcohol in the blood like.

Drink as much, the blood alcohol concentration higher. People often say: there are fewer drunk drinkers, heavy drinkers have not drunk ". The drunk depends on the following factors:

- Before drinking you've eaten? Eat less or more? If you do not eat, the stomach was empty, then you will quickly fall over. Making food in the stomach to the blood alcohol slower moving.

- The way how you drink? Neck or sip? The body of a normal person is capable of absorbing and change wine into another substance - (phenomenon of metabolism) - 9.15 grams of alcohol per hour is equivalent to 340 grams of beer or a glass of wine 142 grams distance or 42 grams of aperitifs.

So you drink 3 glasses of wine in a different time for you to drink 3 glasses of wine but sip during the afternoon.

What kind of wine you drink: vodka containing 50% alcohol, from 3.2 to 5% of beer only wine. Therefore we distinguish heavy alcohol "and wine" light. "Drink" heavy "drunk more quickly.

Carbonate level of alcohol - Champagne with high-quality carbonate, easily absorbed into the body faster than other wines.

Usually body- weight, body-weight of alcohol into the bloodstream faster moving heavier.

201. Advice of people who are earning

Organizing a modern party with wine, toasting each other for blessing are common in doing business.

However, we should pay attention and think about the words of a bank manager reputed as follows: "Do not be unwise to stick with those who drank this glass to the faintest of all the other cups!"

Remember that story doing the "work"! Do not let other people about their bad judgment over the party. Although alcohol is often present in the diplomatic work, but a lot of people have realized that: Do not drink!

If you drink alcohol while communicating, remember that:

- Do not contact job dealing with intoxicated people.

- During the meal, drink is not the principal. Always remember the mission and its purpose at this time to keep the mind sharp.

- If you feel restless, not calm during the meeting, the more it should not drink. Because now you can drink faster and more normal. That makes you more tempered, easily lead to results not to his advantage.

If you're going to a party to talk about his business, should: Drink 1 glass of aperitif. Just click the mouth or drink better.

- If you have champagne, should only sip, slowly.

- When in a party, drink water.

- Avoid supernaculum.

202. When after the drink

Yesterday evening, the cup screwed up this morning because you feel a headache, stomach nausea, ringing in the ears, really unpleasant. Not how to cure that state. However, it may make you uncomfortable abated by.

- Bed rest, as long as possible.

- Avoid bright light, sunlight or a lamp.

- Taking aspirin.

You can avoid this status if:

- During the banquet, eat a lot of fat, meat and cheese can cause you support and heart thumping hangover when served with alcohol.

- Remember the wines such as bourbon, scotch, red wine, peach wine contains substances that have the effect of annoying people drinking gin and vodka longer.

- It's best to never drink too much.

203. Are you addicted?

To know you are drinking for the fun or you're about to addiction, please answer the following questions with "Yes" or "No" and then combine the results again:

1. Do you ever intend to stop drinking one week, but then just stay is a few days?

2. Are you afraid that someone no longer cooperate with you in the business because you know you drink alcohol?

3. Have you ever replace this wine with other wine because they think it less intoxicating new wine better?

4. Last year, you can drink any time during the early morning it?

5. You have wished to be like the guy A, B somehow capable not drink more without getting drunk?

6. Last year a story you met any trouble with the wine or not?

8. Are there times, after a party you went drinking alcohol or intend to go forward because they have not been drinking "was born" in the party?

9. Have you ever declared: "I can stop drinking any time!", But then he does not get drunk?

10. You never have to leave the day before because of excessive drinking or not? '

11. You have been "dull" times because alcohol?

12. Have you ever thought: "this life without alcohol would out what the hell" is not?

If the total number of words, "yes" from 4 or higher, then you need to have a helper to hand out to become a "one wine" and know.

204. Ask anyone to help you quit drinking

The places you can get help with alcoholism are:

1. Psychotherapy - An expert for a detox or for a whole group are very good, to solve the problems of ideological or psychological, the reactions of the body during alcohol withdrawal.

2. Support Team - People who stop drinking can organize a group to help, encourage or solve problems together behalf treacherous during withdrawal.

3. Use herbal - Your doctor may tell you to use disulflram substance, a substance made her uncomfortable when drinking.

4. Rehabilitation Center - is the meeting point of coordination work with hospitals, nursing homes for treatment to help people with alcohol addiction.

5. Family Physicians - Physician specializing in care of the health of your family knows the situation and drink your wine diseases like then. Therefore, he will set out a cure or treatment for alcoholism method gives you a more pragmatic way.

6. The insurer about family issues - Many communities have contact with the insurance company or family services, help clients quit drinking look in the telephone book for the phone number of these organizations.

7. Father religion - Say good intentions "want to quit drinking your 'to help monitor and encourage the local vicar or you're godfather.

205. Teach your children: do not drink

Drinking is not just a matter of adults. In the past, people of young age, especially at the age of nearly mature, also drink, cause very worrying consequences:

- Causing traffic accidents;

- Damage of the family's wealth, there are acts of violence, rogue behavior.

- Educational level low;

- Causing disorder in society;

- Caused problems stress - stress, making the community must find ways to cope.

You need to know about the children in the house had been drinking or not. To educate young people on this issue, the parents have to the descendants imitate:

- Ideally, adults do not drink. Or if taken, must know his keep moderation. Often children of alcoholics also easy to alcoholism than 4 times higher than children who do not drink.

- Always express care, love and concern for our future.

- Note hold gatherings, family vacation, etc. The atmosphere of the family routine and easy to attract children and prevent them from being the influence and activities of the society are not good drag.

- Speak frankly and openly with the children and the harmful effects of alcohol and the opinion of parents of children drinking problem. To prevent problems before they deeply into this matter.

- Tell your child never to her vehicle driver was drunk. Better to wait for parents to pick up or think of another way to get home than to entrust their lives to the death.

206. If you know who are taking sleeping pills overdose, immediately take them to emergency

Horses, Harry, Scag, Junk, Lords, Schoolboy, Morpho, Hocus, Uncie, Powder, Joy, Snow, Miss Em ma, Dollies. Those are the names of the street in the United States having sold narcotics, anesthetics, which everyone knows. In addition, both banned drugs, drugs are classified as heroni, morphine and cocaine.

Users overdose of drugs often have symptoms such as:

- Status abnormal irritation;

- The dull, indifferent to everything around;

- Temperament vagaries;

- Pupils narrowed eyes;

- Skin rash;

- Red nose, nosebleeds;

- Legs, arms have many scars because the drug.

People overdosing, with symptoms such as:

- The pupil eyes narrowed.

- Pale, sweaty.

- Slow pulse

- Shortness of breath

- Convulsions

- Syncope.

If you know who have these symptoms because sedative medications, anesthetics, hypnotics, the birds of prey, to call an ambulance and taken to the hospital or the nearest health center.

207. How to know whether your children commit to drug?

Some parents with older children before sleep should also open eyes to watch the children. Teenage very committed to the wrong thing difficult to imagine. Among the issues to consider is the most dangerous drug problem. Nothing to worry and evening with a son or daughter get involved smoking, drug use.

If there are kids who smoke the drug, the first phenomenon can parents find the clothes, mattresses, blankets our pillows smelled smoke, or a strange odor. They also have the following symptoms:

- Always in need of money, to the extent possible theft.

- There are 1, 2 kids usually meet in a short time (because only with drugs), mood swings, angry or scared easy.

- Eating or sleeping more than usual.

- The rapid weight loss.

- Who looks sullen, disappointed.

- Indifference to everything around, not paying attention to hygiene and clothes, dressing down.

- Concealing everyone in the family of his friends, especially some new friend.

- Knowledge faltering.

If children can see phenomena like this, needless to say frankly to them that they attract parents are suspected drug users. Must calmly explain that they see the harmful effects of alcohol and drugs for human dignity, health and their future.

Drugs can also make them illegal. Must resolutely towards their children about this issue and let us know the program of action of parents and families to prevent and dragged them out of the way drug addiction.

Why should you not smoke marijuana?

In the United States, Marijuana is a drug in the form of tobacco, such as cigarettes, is widely known. It can cause hallucinations smokers, find delight in the cold heart, but everyone and everything around, do whites redness, increased heartbeat, eating more than usual, head dizziness and memory loss in a short time.

The children are often scrambling, caught before, challenge each other attractive are regarded as a mimic of fun like a drink and smoke. What a disastrous mistake for.

Parents need to stop and just tell the children the harm of Msnjuana, such as:

- People who smoke Marijuana and driving and drunk people, prone to accidents.

- Smoking a marijuana by smoking 16 pieces of cigarettes, with declining strength effects.

- With marijauna impair male: sperm count, the number of blood cells, the amount of testosterone is the male sex hormone. Therefore, the phenomenon may lead to weakening or impotence vitality.

- With women, marijauna can cause miscarriage.

- Smokers do Marijauna memory loss, inability to think and comment, tired and dull.

Generally, manjauna harmful to the brain, lungs, heart and all the organs in the body.

The substance is harmful fumes and vapors.

Not only smoke and harmful new drug, but most of the fumes and vapors are not good for human health, especially for children ages 12 and younger, such as coatings, glue, nail polish quality, detergent, adhesive. The plastic vapor inhaling it often:

- Cough, nausea, sneezing, dizziness, hallucinations.

- Children breathing in vapor, toxic fumes may be loss of blood diseases, leukemia and died suddenly.

208. Do not let cocaine enchant you

Before 1970, it was only regarded as a distinct cocaine pharmaceutical capable of sedation, analgesia is very effective. People only think of the advantages of it without thinking much about its harmful effects. Cocaine can make users it sees alertness, euphoria, but gradually become addicted.

Missing cocaine addict disorder both physiological and psychological, can not do anything at all. Previously, when a body part in pain, people use cocaine to relieve pain. Now addicted then, without cocaine, the entire body is in pain. Addicts can chew, injected, inhaled cocaine and depend on it for life.

Use of cocaine overdose, its effects can last from 2 to 4 days, with symptoms: cough, limp or a sudden heart attack. Cocaune first user may be so.

Use of cocaine to:

- Thinking to the harmful effects of cocaine.

- Set the level of cocaine use anywhere, and plans to drop gradually, not any more.

- Do not use cocaine several times a day, or several days.

- Do not hide you and your family about your cocaine. Remember that cocaine is harmful to health, work and relationships of ourselves with others.

If you find yourself or a loved one may be addicted to cocaine, said to a doctor to seek treatment.

209. Be careful when taking valium

Diazepan Valium or sedatives is considered as being normal. But users always be able to get addiction. Users of instant 2, 4 weeks may see the symptoms:

- There frighten, touched;

- Nervous tension, nervousness, palpitations;

- The ability to smell and taste (flavor) decreased;

- Difficulty sleeping;

In summary, your health situation may be worse than before dosing. If you saw it, so to ask the treating physician to take measures to relieve the dose and duration of use.

If you need medication, to avoid addiction, remember:

- Only small doses.

- Do not use more than 3-4 consecutive weeks.

- When you feel the medication is no longer sedative effect, to stop using immediately.

- Use 2 day intervals or in accordance with the instructions of the doctor. They take valium, without using other sedatives.

- Do not drink alcohol while taking the drug

- Women who are pregnant, are pregnant or suspected pregnancy is not intended for medication, valium have a negative impact on the development of the pregnancy.

210. Be careful when using sleeping pills

Few people think we can addict to sleeping pills as well as alcoholism. If you take sleeping pills seamless for 2 weeks you will see the effects as the drug is reduced. For example, you previously had only taken a sleeping pill, this should have 1.5 members, then to 2 tablets ...

Older people, older people need to be more careful when using drugs, because the ability to receive medication in the elderly is lower in middle-aged and young people.

If you may have to phase it is about addiction, you have these symptoms:

- Take the evening before bedtime, exceed 2 weeks.

- Increasingly want higher doses.

- You automatically increase the dose, without a doctor's opinion.

Users overdose of sleeping pills when reaction stammer often slurred, the lethargic, dull, unfocused thinking is, sleep constantly and may die.

Had to take her to the emergency place. If you feel addicted to drugs, tell your doctor need to take measures to stop smoking.

CONCLUSION

Health issues can come to us in many different forms: short-term and chronic, urgent and daily. Fever, aches in head and backbone, runny nose, sore throat, and fatigue - flu symptoms can make you feel so bad that they stop you right from every of your living activities. Unlike the common cold, the flu is a serious respiratory disease that can lead to potentially dangerous complications.

Before a health issue can cause you unnecessary annoyance, you should have a good attention to your health state and good base of health knowledge to forecast the upcoming diseases and avoid them timely or to have proper treatments when it is needed. Whether it's a potential pandemic such as bird flu or an outbreak of hepatitis A, we need to proactively monitor our body's reactions to get the best state of health.

It is clear that no one has all the answers to solve all our health problems, but this project is expected to provide you with some tips at a very basic level that could help you to improve certain health concerns we face almost every day in a more effective way.

Books by KiO Health

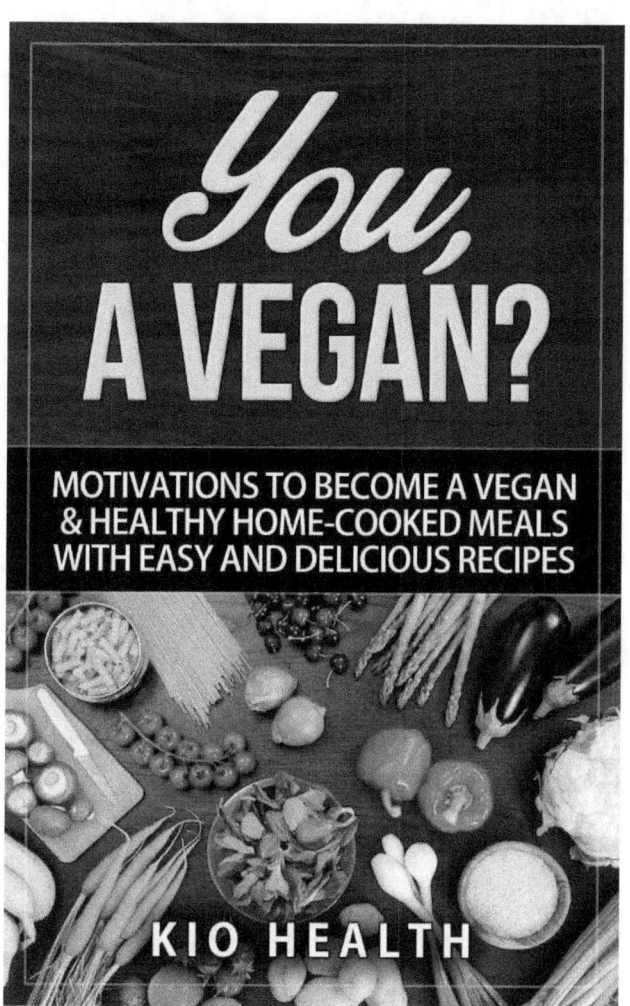